HEALTH & WEIGHT-LOSS
BREAKTHROUGHS 2012

HEALTH & WEIGHT-LOSS BREAKTHROUGHS 2012

FROM THE EDITORS OF 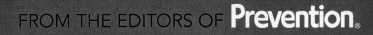Prevention®

RODALE

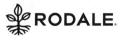

We inspire and enable people to improve their lives and the world around them.

For more of our products, visit prevention.com or call 800-848-4735.

CONTENTS

BONUS

PART 3
FITNESS MOVES

PART 4
NUTRITION NEWS

PART 5
MIND MATTERS

PART 6
BEAUTY BREAKTHROUGHS

INTRODUCTION

LIFE MOVING A LITTLE TOO FAST THESE DAYS? Feel like you can only think in 140-character bursts? We understand!

The irony is that if you take the time to take care of yourself so that you *feel* better, with more energy and less stress, you'll *do* better at work, at home—in life. *Health & Weight-Loss Breakthroughs 2012* will show you how! With the tips, tricks, and techniques in this book, you can improve your health so that you can look, think, feel, *be* better.

Health & Weight-Loss Breakthroughs 2012 is filled with the latest health breakthroughs on weight loss, nutrition, fitness, mind matters, and beauty. Here, you'll find smart strategies to apply these medical breakthroughs to your own life.

In Part 1: Health Breakthroughs, you'll discover the latest amazing innovations that can enhance your health and well-being. First, take our test to determine your "feel age." Then discover the latest pain control breakthroughs, surprising benefits of sex, and why your breakfast cereal might be increasing your risk of cancer.

In Part 2: Weight-Loss Wisdom, you'll discover the latest information about losing weight. Find out how you can eat anything, anywhere, and still lose weight. Learn how to reset your hunger clock. Try an easy-to-use tool, which we bet you've never heard of, to transform your body in 3 short weeks.

Turn to our Bonus Weight-Loss Cookbook for 35 of this year's best *Prevention* recipes. They're delicious, nutritious, and easy to make to boot. Our favorites are the Fall Frittata, Autumn Salad, Mashed Sweet Potatoes with Apple Juice, Pulled Pork Pizza, and of course the Triple Chocolate Cheesecake.

Get movin' and groovin' with Part 3: Fitness Moves. Learn how to walk off weight three times faster. Lose a size this month—without dieting. Build your perfect gym and get into the best shape of your life—without even leaving your comfy home.

In Part 4: Nutrition News, you'll learn how to eat better than ever. First, you'll discover the new power foods and some critical health-boosting nutrients you might be missing. You'll save money by learning about some surprising shelf lives of foods. And you'll get back to basics and simplify your life by eating more natural, wholesome foods.

If you're feeling blue, stressed, or fatigued, check out the new strategies and innovations in Part 5: Mind Matters. You'll discover the long view of a happy life. Learn breakthrough mind games that help your health. And pick up dozens of pillow-tested, all-natural, sound-sleep tricks to help you sleep better—tonight!

You'll look great after following the tips in Part 6: Beauty Breakthroughs. Here's how to get great skin, whether you have a day, a week, or a month. Enjoy 10 foods that rejuvenate skin and deliver important health benefits, too, such as reducing your risk of cancer, heart disease, and diabetes. You *can* eat your way to better-looking skin! And trim away the years with our natural hair makeovers.

We've filled this book with the latest and greatest health and weight-loss news and information. Best wishes for tremendous health and happiness!

Part 1

HEALTH
Breakthroughs

CHAPTER 1

What's Your Feel Age?

You know your real age, but what counts is your "feel age"

Attitude, sense of self, and the state of your emotions all shape your ongoing zest for life. Take our quiz, created by Nicola Gates, a clinical neuropsychologist in Sydney, Australia, to find out your feel age. Then, learn how to maintain your most confident outlook.

THE QUIZ

Relax: There are no right or wrong answers. But what you learn about yourself can help shave years off your feel age. As you answer, keep a tally of the negative numbers and the positive numbers. After you complete the quiz, you'll add the negative scores together and separately total the positives. You'll find out your feel age—and how to adjust it—on page 8. Ready to learn your feel age? Simply turn the page!

1. Do you feel physically strong and capable most days?
   - ❏ Never +2
   - ❏ Rarely +1
   - ❏ Sometimes 0
   - ❏ Often -1
   - ❏ Always -2

2. When you size yourself up against others your age, how often do you feel you're in good (or even better!) shape?
   - ❏ Never +2
   - ❏ Rarely +1
   - ❏ Sometimes 0
   - ❏ Often -1
   - ❏ Always -2

3. Do you see your body as sexy, shapely, attractive—any, or all, of these?
   - ❏ Never +2
   - ❏ Rarely +1
   - ❏ Sometimes 0
   - ❏ Often -1
   - ❏ Always -2

4. Are you at ease shooting off a text message or Twittering?
   - ❏ Never +2
   - ❏ Rarely +1
   - ❏ Sometimes 0
   - ❏ Often -1
   - ❏ Always -2

5. Are you the knowledge-seeking, Google-eyed, curious type?
   - ❏ Never +2
   - ❏ Rarely +1
   - ❏ Sometimes 0

- ❏ Often -1
- ❏ Always -2

6. How often do you feel let down by what your body can achieve?
- ❏ Never -2
- ❏ Rarely -1
- ❏ Sometimes 0
- ❏ Often +1
- ❏ Always +2

7. Whether it's your "muffin top" or your "jelly belly," how often do you negatively rate your body?
- ❏ Never -2
- ❏ Rarely -1
- ❏ Sometimes 0
- ❏ Often +1
- ❏ Always +2

8. How regularly do you wake up feeling more tired or sad than excited and energetic?
- ❏ Never -2
- ❏ Rarely -1
- ❏ Sometimes 0
- ❏ Often +1
- ❏ Always +2

9. As you age, do you feel more confident and optimistic about what the future holds?
- ❏ Never +2
- ❏ Rarely +1
- ❏ Sometimes 0
- ❏ Often -1
- ❏ Always -2

10. Do you draw inspiration and support from your friends?

- ❏ Never +2
- ❏ Rarely +1
- ❏ Sometimes 0
- ❏ Often -1
- ❏ Always -2

11. Do you have friends in every age group, from 18 to 88?

- ❏ Never +2
- ❏ Rarely +1
- ❏ Sometimes 0
- ❏ Often -1
- ❏ Always -2

12. Are you prepared to gracefully accept some aspects of aging?

- ❏ Never +2
- ❏ Rarely +1
- ❏ Sometimes 0
- ❏ Often -1
- ❏ Always -2

13. Do you think getting older means losing your marbles?

- ❏ Never -2
- ❏ Rarely -1
- ❏ Sometimes 0
- ❏ Often +1
- ❏ Always +2

14. Do you get excited about experiencing new things?

- ❏ Never +2
- ❏ Rarely +1
- ❏ Sometimes 0
- ❏ Often -1
- ❏ Always -2

15. Do you feel under siege from minor illness and fatigue?

- ❏ Never -2
- ❏ Rarely -1
- ❏ Sometimes 0
- ❏ Often +1
- ❏ Always +2

16. Do you actively help other people or volunteer for charity?

- ❏ Never +2
- ❏ Rarely +1
- ❏ Sometimes 0
- ❏ Often -1
- ❏ Always -2

17. How often do you feel that these are your best years?

- ❏ Never +2
- ❏ Rarely +1
- ❏ Sometimes 0
- ❏ Often -1
- ❏ Always -2

18. Does your face reveal a happy, no-holds-barred kind of life?

- ❏ Never +2
- ❏ Rarely +1
- ❏ Sometimes 0
- ❏ Often -1
- ❏ Always -2

19. Mirror, mirror . . . do you look older than your age?

- ❏ Never -2
- ❏ Rarely -1
- ❏ Sometimes 0
- ❏ Often +1
- ❏ Always +2

20. Do you often think that getting older is the pits?

- ❑ Never -2
- ❑ Rarely -1
- ❑ Sometimes 0
- ❑ Often +1
- ❑ Always +2

21. Is there meaning and fulfillment in your life?

- ❑ Never +2
- ❑ Rarely +1
- ❑ Sometimes 0
- ❑ Often -1
- ❑ Always -2

22. Socially and politically, do you feel you have some opinions to share?

- ❑ Never +2
- ❑ Rarely +1
- ❑ Sometimes 0
- ❑ Often -1
- ❑ Always -2

What's Your Feel Age?

Add all the negative scores together and, separately, total up the positives. Write down your age. Now subtract the negatives, add the positives, and that's your feel age! It's a score based on your physical confidence, personal development, optimism, and attitude toward aging. Read on to see how you can adjust the dial.

If your feel age is younger than your real age . . . you're the adventurous, positive type; you love life and are young at heart. You feel physically capable. Friends and family draw on your zesty approach to life. "You're aging fabulously," says Nicola Gates. "Maintain your healthy, balanced lifestyle and keep celebrating life." In other words, don't succumb to a funk as the big birthdays—50, 60, 70—roll around. Instead, mark these important milestones by throwing a party! Continue investing your time and energy in doing

WANT TO FEEL EVEN YOUNGER?

We can't change our genetic makeup, but we have a lot of control over daily habits, which go a long way to ensure that we age positively.

HAVE SEX. Couples in their mid-forties who have sex three times a week look up to 12 years younger than those who enjoy intercourse less often, finds one study.

EAT RIGHT. The hearts of women and men who limited their daily calories to 1,400 to 2,000 functioned like those of people 15 years their junior.

DO PUZZLES. Such brain exercises can sharpen your mental abilities so much that your brain will perform like those of folks more than a decade younger.

what you love; the satisfaction will invigorate both you and your close relationships. Stay emotionally intimate with your spouse. A healthy sex life, an active social life, and loads of physical exercise will help keep you sizzling.

If your feel age matches your real age . . . you are balanced, lively, realistic, and curious. You have a strong sense of self that, along with your other strengths, constitutes a great recipe for positive aging. To hold steady at the same feel age for another 5 years, sprinkle your calendar with friendly get-togethers and get an MP3 player or iPod and spend a weekend loading it.

Keep getting the physical workouts you need—at least 30 minutes four or five times a week. And don't pick up any new bad habits, such as settling for inadequate sleep or turning a blind eye to portion control.

If your feel age is older than your real age . . . self-awareness and honesty are two of your strengths, yet it's likely you have some health concerns preventing you from aging in a more positive way. "Make a new beginning. Put the way you see and describe yourself under the microscope and work out how to celebrate who you are," says Gates. Start by writing a list of what you're good at and what you appreciate about yourself. Some traits to consider: creativity, humor, and kindness. Also, boost your exercise to at least 2 hours a week, and organize more face time with friends. "Research shows those who socialize often age better," she says.

CHAPTER 2

Pain Control Breakthroughs

Is your pain treatment hurting? Chronic pain affects millions of Americans and is notoriously tricky to control. Here are some of the most common mistakes pain sufferers make—and the smarter steps that will help you feel better fast

A year after giving birth to her third child, Teresa Shaffer began to feel excruciating pain in her back. An MRI revealed that the cushiony disks in her back were deteriorating, a sign of osteoarthritis, a degenerative joint disease that typically arises much later in life. She was only 24.

"Because I was so young, the doctor didn't believe I had the disease," says Shaffer, now 46. He told her to take OTC pain relievers.

It wasn't until she visited a different doctor that she began to truly get help. He asked if she was depressed (back pain and depression often go hand in hand), prescribed an antidepressant, and referred her for counseling. He sent her for physical therapy and put her on the fentanyl patch, a strong opioid

WHAT'S THE ALTERNATIVE?
THE HERB THAT BEATS BACK PAIN

Ointment with comfrey extract, which has anti-inflammatory properties, helped ease back pain in a recent study. After applying it to sore spots for 5 days, 95 percent of subjects reported improvement, compared with 38 percent in the placebo group. Keep in mind: The herb has alkaloid compounds that can cause liver damage, which is why you should not use it orally. Limit topical use to 10 days or fewer, and don't apply it to broken skin. The study's brand, Kytta-Salbe f, is made by Merck and available in the United States at www.smallflower.com ($17.50 per tube).

for people who need constant medicine. Now she's able to walk for an hour on the treadmill every day.

An estimated 43 million Americans report living with chronic pain, defined as lasting for at least 3 months. Yet experts agree that it's woefully undertreated in our country. Despite breakthroughs in the understanding of pain, few doctors are aware of these advances or are trained in pain management, says Michel Dubois, MD, director of pain education and research at New York University Langone Medical Center.

One major shift in thinking is that chronic pain is now believed to be a disease, not a symptom, and that treating pain is about not simply targeting the source but treating the whole person. As for heart disease or other chronic conditions, there's no magic bullet, so you need to draw on a number of approaches, from exercise and medication to relaxation techniques and talk therapy.

Eliminating pain entirely might not be realistic; what is attainable is to lower it enough to improve your life and do the things you love. If you're making any of the mistakes that follow, we've got the right formula for lasting relief.

MISTAKE: YOU'RE TRYING TO TOUGH IT OUT

One in four pain sufferers waits at least 6 months before seeing a doctor, typically downplaying pain or thinking it'll pass on its own, according to the American Pain Society. And many sufferers self-treat with OTC pain-killers.

Get relief: Seek treatment sooner rather than later. Studies show that the majority of injuries resolve themselves in about 4 weeks, so if yours hasn't—or if your pain is affecting your ability to function—see your doctor. Waiting can wreak havoc on your body and your mind. When pain keeps you from being active, muscles weaken and shrink and joints stiffen, setting you up for further injuries.

Research shows that chronic pain can also lead to depression and even shrink your brain. A study of 26 patients who had back pain for at least 1 year found that they had a 5 to 11 percent loss of brain cells in two areas of the brain—the thalamus and prefrontal cortex—compared with a control group. One explanation is that the neurons are hyperactive for so long that it causes them to break down and die, explains Dr. Dubois. Researchers hypothesize that if the pain persists, it may become less responsive to treatment because of the brain changes.

MISTAKE: YOU'VE SEEN MORE THAN ONE SPECIALIST

In our fragmented health care system, with a specialist for every ailment, it's easy to jump from one doctor to the next. But doctor hopping, experts say, can waste time and money, lead to excessive MRIs and other diagnostic tests, and delay treatment.

Get relief: Find one doctor who can be your point person to coordinate other treatments. Your primary care physician is likely the best person for this. "Just make sure you get a sense that he or she takes your pain seriously, offers you a treatment strategy, and sees you frequently enough to monitor your progress—or refer you to a specialist if your plan is not working," says Russell Portenoy, MD, chairman of the department of pain medicine and palliative care at Beth Israel Medical Center in New York City. That's what Shaffer did. Though her doctor was not fully trained in pain management—and most physicians aren't—"he always did research to find out what my next step should be," she says.

If you've been suffering for months with no improvement, then it may be time to seek out a comprehensive pain management center. (To find one, visit the Web site of the American Academy of Pain Management at www. aapainmanage.org.) If you don't have pain management experts near you, look for a specialist who deals with the source of your pain, such as an orthopedist for back pain or a rheumatologist for arthritis or fibromyalgia.

NATURAL WAYS TO EASE PAIN

Consider these simple—and free—natural pain relief strategies.

BREAK OUT YOUR PHONE. Flip through family photos before an uncomfortable procedure like a mammogram to make it more bearable. Women who viewed pictures of their partners during a lab test reported less pain than those who looked at inanimate objects or strangers. A loving face may spur the release of chemicals that shut down pain-processing areas of the brain.

TAKE DEEP, SLOW BREATHS. Women whose breathing rates slowed by half reported significantly less discomfort during a pain-inducing experiment. Measured breathing helps deactivate your body's fight-or-flight response to pain. It can also be a good distraction—something women who've given birth know well!

MEDITATE OFTEN. Wind down before bed with a few minutes of calm. People who meditate regularly have thicker areas of the cortex, a part of the brain that affects pain sensitivity, than those who don't, found Canadian research. A few days of practice may be enough to boost pain tolerance.

MISTAKE: YOU'RE AFRAID TO EXERCISE

It might be the last thing you feel like doing when you're hurting, but study after study shows that exercise reduces all kinds of pain. It strengthens your muscles and oils your joints, making you less likely to get reinjured. It also releases natural pain-relieving endorphins, which can boost your mood, and it fights the inflammation associated with a number of painful conditions like gout and rheumatoid arthritis.

Get relief: Start slow and easy, especially if you've been sedentary for a few months. Do 5 or 10 minutes of walking or another low-impact activity a couple of times a day if that's all you can do. Swimming or aquatic aerobics, especially in warm water, makes it easier to move, takes pressure off joints, and reduces stiffness and pain.

"The goal is to get you to a comfortable level of functioning," says Judith Turner, PhD, a professor of psychiatry and behavioral sciences at the University of Washington. For people who have fibromyalgia, low- or moderate-intensity activities reduce pain better than high-intensity ones.

A physical therapist can guide you and help lay out a safe plan. But other treatments offered by physical therapists or practitioners, such as ultrasound and electrostimulation, have little evidence to support their effectiveness beyond short-term symptom relief, says Tim Carey, MD, director of the Cecil G. Sheps Center for Health Services Research at the University of North Carolina.

MISTAKE: YOUR INSTINCT IS SURGERY BEFORE THERAPY

Surgery might seem like the most efficient option, but for chronic pain, the research is mixed. Studies show that operating to relieve lower-back pain without any evidence of nerve pressure, for example, might offer minimal, if any, benefit compared with a rehabilitation program—not to mention that it comes with risks.

"The truth is any surgery has a chance of making your pain worse from infection, scarring, and nerve damage," says Dr. Carey.

Get relief: Opt first for pain medications, physical therapy, or exercise. To treat back pain, for example, experts recommend trying a combination of the three for at least 6 months before discussing surgical options. Many people will improve enough to either avoid or no longer be eligible for surgery, says William Abdu, MD, medical director of the Spine Center at Dartmouth-Hitchcock Medical Center. You can also talk with your doctor about trying a shorter, more intensive rehabilitation program.

MISTAKE: YOU'RE WARY OF NARCOTICS

The news is filled with stories about unintentional deaths from pain meds or celebs who became hooked on them, so many pain sufferers prefer to play it safe with OTC pain relievers. Even some physicians avoid narcotics for fear of being punished for overprescribing them. But the reality is, most people in pain aren't going to get addicted to or die from pain meds. And the benefits of taking them are immense. When you're in less pain, you can be more active and speed your recovery.

Get relief: Most doctors start patients on low doses of opioids and require check-in evaluations every 3 or 4 weeks to make sure the medication is working well. If you experience that "drugged" feeling in the beginning, don't worry. It'll go away in a few days as your body adjusts to the medication. Take

---

30-SECOND FOOT PAIN FIX

Are your feet in pain? Stretching can keep your feet healthy and ready to move. For flexible, pain-free arches and toes, do this stretch from Susi Hately, founder of Functional Synergy yoga therapy, every other day.

Kneel on a folded towel; tuck your feet under so you're on your toes. Sit back, with your hips on your heels.

Untuck so the tops of your toes are on the floor, with your feet perpendicular to the floor. Too intense? Lean forward. Hold each stretch for 30 seconds to 2 minutes.

---

the drug only as prescribed. Don't increase the dose or combine it with other types of drugs, such as muscle relaxants or antianxiety drugs, unless you've talked with your doctor.

All that said, there are some people who might be predisposed to addiction. If you've had a problem with alcohol or drugs in the past, you'll have to be monitored even more closely by your doctor. Signs of addiction include feeling compulsive about taking the drug, being unable to control how much you take, and showing no signs of improvement.

MISTAKE: YOU HAVEN'T CONSIDERED NATURAL TREATMENTS

If you can't take pain meds because of side effects or are just looking to enhance their effects, consider alternative treatments. Clinical studies show that acupuncture, for example, relieves osteoarthritis pain, sciatica, and lower-back problems. Rheumatoid arthritis sufferers can benefit from the anti-inflammatory effects of omega-3 fatty acids supplements. According to a large review of recent research, patients who took devil's claw, white willow bark, and cayenne for lower-back pain had more relief than those who took a placebo.

Get relief: Herbal therapies are not without side effects and they may interfere with other medications, so talk with your doctor before taking them. For a science-based primer on top natural pain fighters, go to www. prevention.com and search "natural remedies for pain management."

Numerous studies also show that mental techniques can help ease pain. Start with some simple relaxation techniques: Practice deep breathing and tightening and relaxing different muscles for 15 to 20 minutes every day. A therapist can help you learn other types of relaxation, such as visualization, self-hypnosis, and biofeedback. Ask your doctor for a referral.

MISTAKE: YOU DON'T DISCUSS DEPRESSION

About 54 percent of people with chronic back pain suffer from depression, but only one-third of them take antidepressants, according to a recent study. New brain-imaging research, however, clearly shows that our mental state is intricately tied to how we process—and deal with—pain. Brain scans show that in patients with chronic pain, the parts that light up are involved with emotion, not just sensation.

"It implies that our emotions have a profound influence on how we perceive pain, how much distress it causes, and ultimately how it affects our quality of life," explains Dr. Portenoy.

Get relief: If you feel hopeless, sleep more or less than usual, and gain or lose weight rapidly, you could be suffering from depression. Discuss your symptoms and options with your doctor, who might prescribe an antidepressant, recommend cognitive behavioral therapy (CBT), or even suggest a combination of the two. CBT teaches you how to better cope with and adapt to your pain (and even train your mind to reduce it), which helps lessen the emotional stress that can make the pain feel worse.

"There is more science showing the benefit of cognitive behavioral approaches than there is for most of the drugs for pain," says Dr. Portenoy. In one recent study, patients with depression and pain were randomly assigned to receive antidepressants and, after 3 months, were given six sessions of CBT. A year later, those in the intervention group were significantly less depressed and had less pain than those who were only informed that they had depressive symptoms and should seek advice about treatment.

To find a CBT specialist, visit the National Association of Cognitive-Behavioral Therapists at www.nacbt.org; for psychologists who focus on pain management, check out the AAPM Web site at www.aapainmanage.org.

MISTAKE: YOU DON'T DO YOUR OWN RESEARCH

Doing a little digging on your own behalf might open you up to new treatment options, help you ask more pointed questions, and improve your sense of control over your care. Antonia Kent, 39, injured her back when she was 21 and underwent three failed surgeries before deciding it was time to look into different options herself.

"I went to the library and read about my particular injury and pain treatments," says the teacher from Union, New Jersey. "It made me feel proactive and not a victim of my pain." The research gave her ideas about which doctors to talk to and therapies to try. After her third surgery, she started taking a stronger medication that got her back on her feet. Today she takes a milder medication with herb supplements, and her pain is much better controlled.

Get relief: Research your specific condition on patient advocacy Web sites, such as the American Pain Foundation (www.painfoundation.org). Also consider joining local chronic pain support groups, where you can get doctor recommendations and share ideas about treatments.

You can find tools online as well to help you decide whether to have surgery, take a particular test, or continue with treatment. A good resource: Go to the Dartmouth-Hitchcock Medical Center Web site (www.dhmc.org) and search for Center for Shared Decision Making. There you can download questionnaires or borrow videos to help you weigh risks and benefits.

CHAPTER 3

The Surprising New Benefits of Sex

If you think you can't survive without it, you might be right. Here are seven surprising ways sex can do a body good

You know sex feels good and does wonders for your mood, but did you know that it benefits your health in a number of not-so-obvious ways? The reason, according to scientists, is that during lovemaking, our bodies produce a cascade of hormones (and other biological changes) that can ease pain, lower cancer risk, boost immunity, and even offset menopausal symptoms in women. Taking care of your health has never been so much fun.

SEX REDUCES CHRONIC PAIN

Ladies, next time you have a headache, just say yes. Stimulation of your clitoris and vaginal walls triggers the release of endorphins, corticosteroids, and other natural painkillers. As a result, you'll feel less pain from headaches and sore muscles during sex.

The benefit, which begins before a woman orgasms, can linger for up to 2 days, says Barry Komisaruk, PhD, a Rutgers University psychology professor and coauthor of *The Science of Orgasm*. In his research, he found that women could withstand painful pressure to their fingers while they were stimulated with sex toys; during orgasm, pain tolerance doubled. And self-stimulation through the front wall of the vagina, where some find their G-spot, increases pain tolerance and pain detection thresholds by up to 50 percent, reports Dr. Komisaruk.

SEX LOWERS BREAST CANCER RISK

During arousal and orgasm, levels of "happiness" hormones rise. Two of these—oxytocin and DHEA—might help keep breasts cancer free. One study showed that women who have sex more than once a month have a lower risk of developing breast cancer than those who are less sexually active.

Greek researchers found that men who had at least seven orgasms a month in their fifties had a significantly lower chance of developing male breast cancer.

A SIP OF GREAT SEX

Here's something worth toasting. Italian researchers recently found that women who drink red wine in moderation show higher levels of sexual interest and lubrication than women who drink less or none at all. Researchers believe the combination of antioxidants and alcohol in the red wine may increase the production of nitric oxide, gas that helps artery walls to relax, which increases bloodflow to the genitals. For steamier sessions in the sack, cap your intake at one to two glasses a day; any more may impair your body's sexual response.

DO BIRTH CONTROL PILLS KILL SEX DRIVE?

Not necessarily, says Richard Harkness, a consultant pharmacist and the author of five books on evidence-based natural medicine. Although some research shows that the hormones in birth control pills may in turn depress testosterone levels, thus sapping libido, other findings show that oral contraceptives have no direct effect on a woman's love life. The bad rap might be related to the fact that earlier versions of the Pill contained higher hormone doses that caused more bloating, headaches, nausea, and breast tenderness—all of which could dampen desire—than current formulations. Factors such as stress, relationship issues, and other meds (like antidepressants or high-blood-pressure drugs) affect sex drive more commonly than birth control pills alone. That said, if you've recently switched to the Pill and suspect a related sex drive dip, talk with your doctor about an alternative birth control method. Think it could be drug related? A different medication might be the answer.

IT GIVES YOUR HEART A WORKOUT

Cardiologists rank intercourse as a mild- to moderate-intensity exercise that enhances heart health as well as brisk walking does. As with any workout, the more vigorous you are, the more your heart benefits. The positions you try matter, too; being on top is especially cardiac-friendly because it usually requires more effort. Orgasm delivers a bonus: At your peak moment, your heart rate may hit 110 beats per minute, comparable to what you might achieve when walking quickly or jogging.

IT PROTECTS THE PROSTATE

Catholic priests have an elevated chance of dying of prostate cancer, and studies point to celibacy as a factor. In 2003, research on middle-aged Australian men found that those who averaged at least four ejaculations a week had a one-third lower chance of developing prostate cancer than those who had fewer.

"When you drain the pipes, as it were, you have less clogging," says Irwin Goldstein, MD, head of San Diego Sexual Medicine at Alvarado Hospital. Though the results of the study were clear, the reasons they occurred were not, says Dr. Goldstein, who calls for more research.

IT LOWERS STRESS

Got a big presentation coming up at work? A 2005 study found that men and women who had engaged in intercourse in the 2 weeks before a stressful day had an easier time while doing public speaking and some verbal arithmetic. During their presentations, their systolic blood pressure (the first

THREE GET-CLOSER COUPLE STRETCHES

Moves designed for two can build trust and strengthen your relationship while helping you both to relax and increase flexibility, says John Friend, founder of Anusara yoga, who came up with these stretches. You can practice them daily, holding each pose for 30 to 60 seconds and alternating positions as you go.

UPPER-BACK AND SHOULDER STRETCH: Face each other and hold each other's wrists. Step apart, bend your knees, and squat down, drawing your hips away from one another. Gaze at the floor and keep your neck relaxed.

LOWER-BACK RELEASE: Lie faceup with your partner holding your ankles. Relax, keeping your hips on the floor, as he or she gently swings your legs side to side in an arc pattern for 30 to 60 seconds.

CHEST STRETCH: Stand with your back to your partner, with your arms at your sides, and your palms forward. Have your partner hold your arms just above your wrists. Lean forward as he or she steps back and gently pulls your arms up.

number in a blood pressure reading) increased less and then dropped back to its normal level at a faster rate than that of people who had no sexual relations or had other forms of sex, including noncoital interactions or masturbation.

One theory about why this occurs is that intercourse requires more complex brain activity; another idea is that it stimulates a number of important nerves not triggered during other sexual activity.

IT REVS UP YOUR IMMUNE SYSTEM

Research from Wilkes University showed that college students who engaged in sex once or twice a week had 30 percent higher levels of infection-fighting antibodies than did their abstinent classmates. In 2004, German scientists observed similar results: Blood tests showed that arousal and orgasm in men increased levels of certain pathogen-fighting white blood cells. The effect is

71 THE PERCENTAGE OF PEOPLE WHO ALWAYS LOOK FOR WAYS TO INCREASE PLEASURE IN BED, ACCORDING TO A TROJAN SURVEY

SEX THAT TRULY SATISFIES

New lingerie isn't the only way for women to turn up the heat. In fact, the most intimate and content couples share some surprisingly simple habits. Here are four signs you're among them.

YOU LIKE SLOW HANDS. Very orgasmic women tend to take their time in the sack and have a more diverse sexual repertoire, says Debby Herbenick, PhD. Her research shows that close couples will do four or five different things in bed (touching, oral sex, various positions) instead of just one or two.

YOU EAT LIKE APHRODITE. Women with type 2 diabetes who ate Mediterranean-style diets reported more sexual satisfaction—as well as lower body mass indexes and less depression, according to a recent study. These confidence boosters, along with improved circulation, mean eating like a Greek can help all women. Say *opa!*

YOU SWEAT OUTSIDE YOUR BEDROOM. Exercise-loving women had better clitoral blood flow (read: more-intense orgasms) than couch potatoes did, a Turkish study found. The mood boost from a good, sweaty jog may also make you feel more desirous—and desirable—in bed.

YOUR HUSBAND SWEATS, TOO. Moderately active men (who completed about 30 minutes of cardio 4 days a week) were 65 percent less likely to have erectile dysfunction than those who rarely hit the gym.

comparable to that of other stress-busting activities, such as exercise and listening to music, which also boost secretion of certain proteins that defend the body against infection.

IT DEFEATS MENOPAUSAL DRYNESS

Scientists in New Jersey found that postmenopausal women who had sexual relations more than 10 times a year had less evidence of vaginal atrophy than those who reported less frequent sex. That's a sign of healthy tissues, says Sandra Leiblum, PhD, a New Jersey sex therapist who helped conduct the study. Arousal brings blood to the vagina, which delivers nutrients and oxygen. Keep using this part of your body, and you'll help prevent the tissue from becoming thinner and less elastic as you age, so intercourse can remain comfortable and pleasurable.

CHAPTER 4

The Cancer Promoter in Your Breakfast Cereal

Research links too much folic acid—a staple in multivitamins, as well as cereal and bread—to colon, lung, and prostate cancers. What news about this B vitamin means to you

Chances are, you started your day with a generous helping of folic acid. For more than a decade, the government has required enriched grains—most notably white flour and white rice—to be fortified with folic acid, the synthetic form of the B vitamin folate. Many food manufacturers take it further, giving breakfast cereals, nutrition bars, and beverages a folic acid boost, too.

The extra nutrient isn't meant for you, though. It's added to protect fetuses from developing rare but tragic birth defects. The fortification effort appears successful: Since 1998, the number of these birth defects dropped by about 19 percent. But for women past the years of having children, as well as for men of any age, unnatural dosages of this nutrient don't seem to be helpful—and might even be harmful. Indeed, many scientists have grown increasingly concerned about mounting research—including a study published in the *Journal of the American Medical Association*—suggesting that all the extra folic acid might increase your odds of developing cancer.

"The more we learn about folic acid, the more it's clear that giving it to everyone has very real risks," says folic acid researcher A. David Smith, PhD, professor emeritus of pharmacology at the University of Oxford in England.

If there's a nutrient it's easy to overdose on, it's folic acid. The vitamin is all around us, slipped into the cereal we eat for breakfast, the bread we eat for lunch, the energy bars we snack on, and the supplements that more than one-third of us take regularly. Women are supposed to get 400 micrograms a day, the amount that protects fetuses. Some cereals, though, contain more or have a serving size that makes it easy to pour a double dose. Add to that a vitamin washed down with your vitamin-fortified drink, and you might get a megadose before walking out the door.

THE FOLIC ACID FALLOUT

The risk experts worry about most: colon cancer. In 2009, health officials in Chile reported that hospitalization rates for colon cancer among men and women age 45 and older more than doubled in their country since fortification was introduced in 2000.

In 2007, Joel Mason, MD, director of the Vitamins and Carcinogenesis Laboratory at Tufts University School of Medicine, described a study of the United States and Canada suggesting that rates of colon cancer rose—following years of steady decline—in the late 1990s (around the time our food began being fortified). Better screening or an aging population could not explain the difference, which amounts to an additional 15,000 cases of cancer per year in the United States alone between 1996 and 2000, according to Dr. Mason's calculations.

"It's a critical enough issue that it can't be ignored," he says.

Other research links high doses to lung and prostate cancers. In one study conducted in Norway, which doesn't fortify foods, supplementation with 800 micrograms of folic acid (plus B_{12} and B_6) daily for more than 3 years raised the risk of developing lung cancer by 21 percent. Another, in which men took either folic acid or a placebo, showed those consuming 1,000 micrograms of folic acid daily had more than twice the risk of prostate cancer. And a new worry recently came to light when scientists discovered the liver has limited ability to metabolize folic acid into folate—which means any excess continues circulating in the bloodstream.

"Unlike folate, folic acid isn't found in nature, so we don't know the effect of the excess," says Dr. Smith.

THE FOLIC ACID PARADOX

Extra folic acid might make sense for all adults (and not just women of childbearing age) if it kept common problems like heart attack, stroke, or age-related memory decline at bay. However, those hoped-for benefits are still in question. We all need the natural folate found in leafy greens, orange juice, and other foods, and diets high in these foods are perfectly healthy. Many researchers, though, believe that folic acid may be both friend and foe.

When cells in the body are healthy, folate helps shepherd along the normal replication of DNA. But when cells are malignant or in danger of becoming so—and as many as half of adults older than 60 could already have precancerous colon polyps, while most middle-aged men have precancerous cells in their prostates—animal studies suggest excess folate in the form of folic acid may act like gas on the fire.

The research is fueling fierce debate in other countries about the wisdom of fortifying the food supply. After 2 years of public hearings, a British government advisory panel recommended in October 2009 that the United Kingdom proceed with mandatory fortification. In contrast, that same year health officials in New Zealand abruptly delayed that country's plans to begin mandatory fortification of bread products.

STAY IN THE SAFE RANGE

"If you're eating a balanced diet and not taking a multivitamin, you're probably fine," says Karin Michels, ScD, PhD, an associate professor in the department of epidemiology at Harvard School of Public Health.

But if you pop supplements and eat a lot of cereal, a lot of bread, and a lot of white rice, you might want to rethink your consumption of folic acid. If it's not possible for you to become pregnant, lowering your intake to 400 micrograms won't hurt and might help save your life. Here's how to do it.

Go natural. Continue to eat as many foods as you want that contain natural folate (leafy greens, citrus fruits, lentils, and dried beans). You can't OD that way.

BIG DOSE, BIG RISK

The following nutrients also should be consumed with caution.

VITAMIN A: Volunteers taking a 5,000 IU supplement of A—or more than 1.5 times the Daily Value of 3,000 IU—increased their risk of stroke and overall mortality in recent research. Equally sobering: A 2007 review of all recent vitamin A studies linked excess amounts of the nutrient to a 16 percent increase in the risk of dying prematurely.

VITAMIN E: About one-quarter of adults over age 60 take high doses of E, which research links to a shorter life span, blood thinning, and a higher risk of lung cancer. The American Heart Association warns that the small amounts in multivitamins are fine, but more than 400 IU daily can increase the risk of early death.

IRON: Before menopause, women need about 18 milligrams of iron daily to prevent anemia. After menopause, they require only about 8 milligrams. Yet cereals, bread, rice, and pasta are often fortified—making it easy to get more without realizing it. Studies show that lowering iron levels reduces the risk of new cancers and cancer mortality. The upshot: Iron supplements are necessary only if prescribed by your doctor.

Read labels. Cereals vary wildly in the amounts of folic acid they contain, and you can probably figure that you're getting more than the label says. One study of the 29 most popular cereals found that the actual level of folic acid and iron was up to three times higher than the amount listed. Check your sports drink, too. Many contain folic acid.

Switch to noninstant oatmeal. It isn't usually fortified, unlike other breakfast cereals.

Go whole grain. Choose whole grain flour, bread, cereal, pasta, and rice. Whole grain foods aren't required to be fortified. As a result, 1 cup of whole wheat flour has only about 50 micrograms of folic acid, while the same amount of refined flour contains almost 400 micrograms. If your bread or cereal is made with whole grain flour, that should be the first ingredient listed.

Rethink that multivitamin. A recent CDC study discovered that half of supplement users who took supplements with more than 400 micrograms of folic acid exceeded 1,000 micrograms per day of folic acid. Most supplements pack 400 micrograms. If you take a multi as insurance, ask your doctor whether individual supplements (of vitamin D and calcium, for instance) may be smarter.

CHAPTER 5

Clean *and* Green

Environmentally friendly household cleaners may not be as safe or as healthy as they claim. Here's what the experts say

A spick-and-span house used to involve a broom, a bucket, and bleach. Times have changed. Now products need to be safe for you and safe for the environment—but still get the job done.

Many people are willing to pay a premium for all three; sales of green cleaning products have skyrocketed 35 percent recently. But are they worth the price—and are they as healthy as they promise to be? In some cases, the answer is no. Here, our experts answer your questions about labels and claims on ecoproducts so you can keep your home clean and green.

ARE ALL GREEN CLEANERS SIGNIFICANTLY BETTER FOR ME OR THE PLANET?

Not necessarily, says Alexandra Gorman Scranton, director of science and research for Women's Voices for the Earth. That's because there is little federal regulation around using the terms *green* or *natural* or even *organic* as a selling point, she explains: "As a result, a manufacturer might market cleaning products as healthier, while still using toxic chemicals, and it's totally legal."

So while green cleaners might contain some healthier ingredients or be a little less toxic to the environment, without anyone regulating the term, companies can make misleading claims that are vague and unsubstantiated. For example, Simple Green's all-purpose cleaner bills itself as nontoxic, but it contains 2-butoxyethanol, a chemical linked in high amounts to red blood cell damage and reproductive problems in animal studies.

WHICH PRODUCTS ARE GOOD AND WHICH AREN'T?

Certain manufacturers and brands—such as ECOS, Method, Clorox Green Works, and SC Johnson's Nature's Source—are putting real muscle behind their green claims, says Stephen Ashkin, executive director of the Green Cleaning Network, a nonprofit that works to educate consumers and institutions about green cleaning. Some are replacing toxic surfactants—the chemicals that help separate dirt from a surface—with healthier, more biodegradable versions. Others are using fewer phthalates, compounds linked to reproductive problems and that are used to add fragrances to cleaning products.

Some major agencies, such as the EPA, also set criteria and certify cleaning products as healthier. The EPA's program Design for the Environment (DfE), for example, requires a scientific review team to screen each ingredient for health and environmental effects and will label a product with a DfE certified logo only if it contains ingredients that pose the least concern among chemicals in their class. Other independent certifying agencies, including Green Seal and EcoLogo, require products to be free of carcinogens and toxins linked to gene mutations, as well as meet certain environmental standards for biodegradability.

DO GREEN CLEANERS WORK AS WELL AS TRADITIONAL ONES?

Experts agree that most of them actually do. Plus, all three major certifying organizations—Green Seal, DfE, and EcoLogo—set performance standards, too, which a product must meet in order to be certified. Some green cleaners can disinfect, as well. The most common ingredients used in green sanitizing products are hydrogen peroxide, citric acid, and lactic acid, which are all considered safer antimicrobials.

HOW CAN I SHOP GREEN?

Step one is to avoid or at least minimize your use of products labeled with the words *warning, poison, flammable,* or *corrosive*—terms that suggest the use of harmful ingredients. Here are guidelines to help you choose a safer product.

Look for green-certified logos on the label. Along with the EPA's DfE label (which you'll find on such brands as Seventh Generation, Earth Choice, and the Martha Stewart Clean product line), Green Seal logos can be found on 29 household cleaners, including Simoniz's Green Scene, Simple Green's Naturals line, and Sustainable Earth cleaners by Staples. In addition, EcoLogo supports such brands as EnviroCare and Nattura.

Skip aerosol sprays. They often contain volatile organic compounds (VOCs), which emit unhealthy gases into the air.

Choose fragrance-free cleaners. Delivering a scent can take a bunch of chemicals, many of which can irritate skin or lungs and may be deemed toxic or hazardous by the EPA.

WHAT ARE THE HEALTHIEST HOME CLEANERS?

DIY cleaners can be the greenest option, according to Alexandra Gorman Scranton of Women's Voices for the Earth, because you can control the ingredients and make sure they're nontoxic.

For cutting boards and countertops: Use vinegar, a nylon scrubbing pad, and water. That's all you need to remove the bacterial film that even strong disinfectants have trouble penetrating, says Allen Rathey, president of the Healthy House Institute.

"Just make sure the water is hot. The heat helps dislodge the foodborne pathogens. And give it a good scrubbing to finish the job," he says. Run porous

(continued on page 40)

GO GREEN, NOT BROKE

The steep prices on some eco cleaners and organic sheets can make green living seem like a luxury few can afford. But if you consider the surprising range of household items that contain dangerous toxins—which scientists say could lead to allergic reactions, thyroid disorders, even cancer—going green starts to sound as much a health priority as an environmental one.

The good news is that you can get many of those benefits with just a few key changes. The following guide will help you decide which areas and items in your home are worth the extra money to buy organic, and which conventional versions are just as good for your body, your wallet, and the planet.

Bedroom

WORTH IT: ORGANIC MATTRESS. Conventional mattresses are laced with chemicals that protect against moisture, fire, and pests. But some of those chemicals create fumes that lead to respiratory problems in mice, says a study in the *Archives of Environmental Health.*

"Since you spend so much of your life with your body pressed against your mattress, an organic one is a great health investment," says Jennifer Taggart, an environmental attorney and consultant and author of *Smart Mama's Green Guide.* "Look for naturally flame-retardant materials like wool, latex, and cocoa husks." Queen-size mattresses from the companies Taggart prefers—OrganicPedic and Naturepedic—start at $1,200, but it's a smart splurge for your health.

PROBABLY NOT: ORGANIC SHEETS AND PAJAMAS. Though insecticides used in conventional cotton production are hard on the planet, they pose little risk to consumers.

"You don't get much, if any, pesticide exposure through clothing or cotton home items," says Rebecca Sutton, a senior scientist for the Environmental Working Group. So you could save for an organic mattress rather than spend on "green" sheets. As for bamboo textiles, last year the Federal Trade Commission charged four manufacturers with falsely claiming their products were ecofriendly. Skip bedding labeled no iron, stain-resistant, or permanent press, as it often has harmful chemicals.

Lawn Care

WORTH IT: EARTH-FRIENDLY FERTILIZER. Many conventional fertilizers are full of heavy metals, which can cause cancer and birth defects, says a 2001 analysis by the California Public Interest Research Group. Plus, they're often prepackaged with a weed-killing pesticide—usually 2,4-D, a chemical cousin of Agent Orange. Given the risks, the added cost for organic fertilizer is worth it.

Plus, "you don't have to apply it as often, and eventually might not have to at all, because it enriches the soil, which chemical fertilizers don't," says Paul Tukey, author of *The Organic Lawn Care Manual* and founder of SafeLawns.org. "Look for a fertilizer derived from plants like alfalfa or seaweed or from bone or fish meal."

Three brands he recommends: Fire Belly Organic Lawn Care, Bradfield Organics, and Dr. Earth.

PROBABLY NOT: ORGANIC COMPOST. If you don't have the space to make compost, you can purchase it, but you don't need organic.

"Regular compost is more than adequate to promote healthy lawns," says Kathy Sargent-O'Neill, a landscape designer and board member of the Ecological Landscaping Association, who differentiates "regular" from the costlier, pesticide-free compost best used for growing organic food crops. "It still feeds the good microscopic critters and keeps grass healthy and green," says Tukey. Just avoid any compost made of "biosolids," which can be a nice way of saying "sewage" and may contain chemicals, he adds.

Green Cleaners

WORTH IT: GREEN LAUNDRY DETERGENT. Switching to certain green cleaners offers great heath benefits.

"Even healthy adults heavily exposed to conventional cleaning products are at greater risk of developing asthma," says Sutton. "We don't even know what's in most of these things because manufacturers don't have to list ingredients."

(continued)

Although eco laundry detergent is pricey, it's especially worth the expense. A 2008 study found that a big-brand conventional detergent had 13 VOCs, five of which are deemed toxic hazards by the EPA. "Plus, many mainstream detergents have chemical scents and optical brighteners, which can irritate skin," says Taggart.

PROBABLY NOT: GREEN DISH DETERGENT. Paying extra for green dishwasher soap is less worth it from a health perspective, notes Taggart. "Unless your machine is malfunctioning, there's little chance of a conventional detergent leaving toxicants on dishes," she says. "Some may contain synthetic fragrance, and inhaling it can expose you to hormone-disrupting phthalates, but it's a relatively small exposure."

cutting boards or those with deep grooves through the dishwasher once a week; the moist heat can destroy lingering germs.

For toilets and bathtubs: Use baking soda and vinegar. Sprinkle a generous amount of baking soda in your bowl or tub and scrub with a brush. To eliminate germs or mold, spray a 10 percent vinegar/90 percent water solution on the surface of your toilet or bathtub; let it sit for at least 30 minutes before rinsing with water.

Stubborn stains might require a commercial cleaner, which can be toxic. If you use such products, open the window or turn on a fan to ventilate the room, and wear gloves as well as protective goggles or glasses to shield your eyes from fumes or splashes.

For mirrors and glass: Use vinegar and water. Spray a solution of 10 percent vinegar/90 percent water and wipe with a clean cloth (preferably a microfiber one, available at such stores as Home Depot and Walmart) to remove oil films, dirt, and dust. Add a dab of dish soap for jobs on windows that involve removing heavy dirt.

For furniture: Use a microfiber cloth and water. To remove dust from surfaces, lightly dampen a microfiber cloth and wipe. If you want the surface to have a slight shine, follow up with a regular cloth dabbed with olive or pure lemon oil. Don't use microfiber with the oil.

HOW CAN I GO GREEN IN THE LAUNDRY ROOM?

While you might be a pro at sorting delicates from dishrags and fighting stains to the death, a few missteps can leave you more susceptible to germs, allergy attacks, skin rashes—even cancer. To help boost your family's health, adopt the following laundry room habits.

To protect against germs, empty the washer ASAP. Bacteria flourish in wet areas, so take clothes out within 30 minutes of a completed cycle. If they sit for an hour, rewash the load. But wouldn't just-laundered clothes be germ free, you wonder? Not necessarily, says Charles Gerba, PhD, professor of environmental microbiology at the University of Arizona. These days, many people are trying to save energy and money by washing with cold water, but harmful bacteria can easily survive in it, explains Dr. Gerba, whose research found that 25 percent of home washing machines contain fecal bacteria. Although the strains of *E. coli* found were fairly harmless, their presence alone indicates that bacteria and viruses can linger on laundry, he says.

Though Dr. Gerba recommends using hot water to kill germs, cold is better for energy bills—and the planet. To help protect your family, don't overload the washer, so detergent can penetrate all the fabric. Also, wash your hands after removing wet clothes so you don't spread lingering germs. The dryer's heat will kill most of the remaining bugs.

Wash undergarments separately. Not surprisingly, the primary source of fecal bacteria in a washer is underwear. It's best to do undies in a separate cycle, with hot water and regular or color-safe bleach, suggests Dr. Gerba. And once a week, run an empty cycle with only a cup of bleach. "That prevents bacteria from hanging out in the drum," he adds.

Wash bedding in hot. Unsavory as it sounds, your sheets and pillowcases house legions of dust mites that dine on the skin cells you shed at night. Dust mites are the most common cause of year-round allergy symptoms. They live in clothes and carpeting, but their highest concentrations are in beds. To alleviate symptoms, it's most important to wash your bedding weekly in hot water (set at a minimum of 130°F), says Robert Weitz, a microbiologist in Stamford, Connecticut.

"If you wash with cold or warm, you're just giving them a nice swim," he says. "And the dryer alone isn't hot enough to kill them."

Air out your washer. Mold spores are always present in the air to some degree, but when they find a wet surface (say, the inside of a washer), they can settle in and multiply. Exposure to mold can cause congestion, itchy eyes, and wheezing. If you're asthmatic or allergic, they can trigger an attack. To prevent mold from growing in your machine and then transferring to your clothes, when you finish your laundry, prop the washer door open to air it out and dry off any visible rubber parts. Be extra diligent with front loaders. They use rubber gaskets to seal the water inside, and mold often grows on them, says Weitz. Another tip: "Buy HE, or high efficiency, detergent," he adds. "It makes less suds than regular kinds, leaving behind less moisture."

Ventilate the room. Moist heat from the dryer can keep humidity levels high, which creates ripe conditions for mold to grow. Leave a window open or turn on a fan when the dryer is running, and check dryer hoses.

"If the vent to the outside comes loose, moisture can get trapped in the wall, and mold can grow," Weitz says.

Choose unscented soaps. You might love clothes that smell like flowers or fresh rain, but it takes a cocktail of chemicals to deliver those scents—chemicals that can irritate your skin, or worse. Researchers at the University of Washington analyzed a popular detergent and found that it emitted 13 VOCs, five of which are regulated as toxic or hazardous by the EPA.

"Often, laundry products can contain hazardous chemicals such as neurotoxins and carcinogens," says study author Anne Steinemann, PhD, professor of civil and environmental engineering at the university. "Exposure to them can cause migraine headaches and asthma attacks."

The kicker: Many of these chemicals aren't related to the detergents' cleansing agents but instead to the fragrances they're scented with. It's best to choose ones free of perfumes and dyes rather than ones merely labeled "unscented." "Unscented may mean a masking agent was used to cover up the detergent aroma, but harmful agents can remain," says Dr. Steinemann. And according to her latest research, laundry detergents with natural or organic scents can be just as toxic as the regular ones.

Toss dryer sheets. They emit chemicals also regulated as toxic and can cause breathing difficulties and irritated skin, says Dr. Steinemann. Liquid fabric softeners can have the same effect.

Instead of dryer sheets, try PVC-free plastic dryer balls (available at Amazon.com). They help more air pass between clothes to cut down on static cling. As a softener, add $\frac{1}{2}$ cup of baking soda to the rinse cycle of your wash.

CHAPTER 6

Better Air, Better Health

Poor indoor air quality can trigger allergies, irritate your lungs, even raise your risk of cancer—and it's now more common than you think. Here's how to keep it clean

Worried about indoor air pollution? You might want to take a deep breath (or not). The EPA says the air in most homes is two to five times more contaminated than the air outdoors.

And it's getting worse. In our zeal to make homes more energy efficient, we've created spaces sealed so tightly that there can be a buildup of fumes (like volatile organic compounds, or VOCs, found in thousands of household products) and biological irritants (such as mold and dust mites).

"The air in your house contains pollen, mold, and ozone that leach in from the outdoors, as well as pet dander and pollutants from household cleaning products," says Ted Myatt, ScD, a senior scientist at the consulting firm Environmental Health and Engineering, Inc.

To make matters worse, come winter, weatherproofing combined with heated, dry air can boost indoor pollution levels higher by sealing in airborne toxins and lowering levels of humidity. The combination of the two can pose an even greater risk.

"Exposure to indoor pollution is associated with allergies, severe asthma, hospitalizations for cardiovascular and respiratory disease, and even heart attacks," Dr. Myatt says.

While we know bad air is tough on people with allergies and asthma, it poses threats to all of us. VOCs cause headaches and fatigue, and radon (a naturally occurring radioactive gas found in many homes) is the second-leading cause of lung cancer.

The good news is that you don't need to spend big bucks to clean the air in your home.

"Many air-quality problems can be addressed with a few low-cost, commonsense solutions, like proper ventilation," says Laureen Burton, a chemist and toxicologist with the EPA.

Considering we spend about 60 percent of our lives in our homes, it's time to clear the air. Here are simple, budget-friendly strategies to clear the air and breathe easier.

TWO WORTH-IT EXPENSES

LOW-VOC PAINT. Your walls are a leading source of these harmful compounds because paint continues to "off-gas" up to a year after it dries, say some experts. Try Benjamin Moore's Natura, for about $50 a gallon.

HEPA VACUUM CLEANER. Short for *high efficiency particle accumulator*, HEPA filters catch virtually all particles that are at least 0.3 micrometer in size. (Otherwise, those tiny pollution particles just float right back into your living room.) Though status brands such as Dyson (which range from $300 to $900) and Miele (from $350 to $1,100) have devoted followings, other companies like Bissell and Eureka sell good ones for $200 or less.

30 THE PERCENTAGE IMPROVEMENT IN FEELINGS OF FATIGUE AMONG WORKERS WHO ADDED PLANTS TO THEIR OFFICES, ACCORDING TO THE AGRICULTURAL UNIVERSITY OF NORWAY

FREE!

Open the windows. Bringing in cleaner outdoor air is the easiest way to dilute the contaminated air in your home. Do it for 10 to 15 minutes a day—unless you live next to a factory, within one-third of a mile of an interstate, or near another potential pollution source, says Jennifer Taggart, an environmental lawyer and author of *Smart Mama's Green Guide.* In those cases, the air outside may be worse. Also, skip it on high-pollen-count days or when it's very humid outside, which can raise the risk of mold.

Vacuum slowly. Dust is a leading source of air pollution because it absorbs toxic gases, including VOCs and radon, says Mark Sneller, PhD, a microbiologist and author of *Greener Cleaner Indoor Air: A Guide to Healthier Living.*

"Vacuuming slowly and methodically captures the most dust," he says. "The faster you go, the more dust you'll raise, which defeats the purpose." Vacuum at least twice a week, he recommends, and step outside to empty the vacuum cleaner bag. That's because bacteria can multiply 100-fold inside a vacuum, says Charles Gerba, PhD, a professor of environmental microbiology at the University of Arizona.

"When you empty the bag, it may release a big cloud of *E. coli* and salmonella into the air," Dr. Gerba says.

Run the bathroom fans. The vents draw moist air out, reducing the risk of mold development. Breathing in mold spores can cause coughing, chest tightness, and itchy eyes; if you're asthmatic or allergic, they can trigger an attack, reports the Centers for Disease Control and Prevention. Run fans whenever you are showering or using products that contain fragrances or vapors, such as nail polish or hair spray, says Dr. Sneller.

(continued on page 50)

WINTERTIME AIR FIXES

Open a window. Sure, that's a great idea when it's 69 degrees outside and sunny. But what about in the middle of winter, when your house is sealed up against the driving rains and howling winds? Here's how to keep your air clearer, even when it's cold outside.

CRACK A WINDOW. Opening up windows when it's freezing outside sounds, well, cold (and costly). But sealing a house too tightly doesn't allow the entry of new oxygen or the escape of carbon dioxide that you exhale. As a result, your body doesn't get the amount of oxygen it needs, and you end up feeling tired and lethargic, explains Matthew Waletzke, a certified building biology consultant on Long Island, New York. He adds, "Oxygen levels can be especially low in a sealed bedroom after a night's sleep."

Open your bedroom windows for 5 to 10 minutes after you wake up in the morning and again before you climb into bed at night; this is enough time to let carbon dioxide out and oxygen in without chilling the rest of your house.

CLEAN UP WHAT YOU BRING DOWN. Dragging winter blankets out of the attic and lugging decorations up from the basement stirs up dust, triggering allergy symptoms such as itchy eyes, wheezing, and congestion, says James Sublett, MD, chief of pediatric allergy at the University of Louisville School of Medicine.

Take boxes outdoors to wipe off the dust, then wipe them down (along with what's inside) before you bring them back in and plop them in the front hall. Wash any blankets or linens in hot water before you use them (same goes for any winter clothes that can go in the washing machine). You can also put on an N95 dust respiratory mask (available at drugstores) before you head to the attic or basement, Dr. Sublett says. It'll shield you from 95 percent of airborne particles that set off sneezing fits, but you'll probably still want to dust off boxes if you plan on taking off the mask.

USE COMMON (CANDLE) SENSE. Scented candles, especially the industrial strength (and size) that many people light, give off more than fragrance. Studies show they produce tiny bits of pollution known as particulates that can inflame the respiratory tract and aggravate asthma, Dr. Sublett says. This is especially true if some of the dust you kicked up unearthing Grandma's decorations is still floating around.

"Allergens like dust can hitch a ride on particulates, enter deep into your lungs, and make breathing more difficult," he explains.

Stop burning candles, especially the ones inside large jars, which tend to send even more particulates into the air, says Jeffrey May, principal scientist at May Indoor Air Investigations in Tyngsborough, Massachusetts, and author of *My House Is Killing Me!* If you can't give up the candle habit, choose unscented tapered candles, and place them far from vents and other air sources.

TURN OFF VENTILATION FANS. Exhaust fans work by sending the stale indoor air outside and replacing it with fresh air. However, running powerful fans such as commercial-size kitchen fans, large exhaust fans, or bathroom fans all at once (especially for an extended period of time) can redirect exhaust gases that may include deadly carbon monoxide fumes produced by gas or oil heaters back into the house instead of up and out the flue, explains Max Sherman, PhD, a senior scientist at Lawrence Berkeley National Laboratory.

Turn exhaust fans off as soon as they've done their job, or consider replacing a manual switch with a timer to limit unnecessary use. Install carbon monoxide detectors as well. They're just as important as fire detectors.

REPLACE FILTHY FILTERS. If your home has dry air, the upside is that it makes it difficult for mold to grow. But existing mold from damp basements and lingering spores in air-conditioning systems can become airborne (and stay there) if all the windows are closed, May says. Mold can irritate your eyes, cause congestion, and worsen existing respiratory problems.

Change your heating system filters every 3 months, Dr. Sublett says. Filters act like armed guards, holding hostage pollutants that feed mold—such as human skin cells, pollen, and pet dander—so they can't escape into your indoor air. May recommends a filter with a minimum efficiency reporting value (MERV) rating of at least 8. Check the packaging. And have a professional service your heating system annually. Summer may be the best time. That way you can fix problems before you need to turn on the heat.

Clean furnace and AC filters. If they're dirty or damaged, they don't work. Follow the recommended maintenance schedule for heating and air-conditioning systems. Generally, filters should be checked about four times a year, says the American Lung Association.

Forget the fireplace. Burning wood emits harmful toxins that worsen breathing problems, which can lead to heart and lung disease and even early death, according to the American Lung Association. In San Francisco between November and February, wood burning contributes to 33 percent of fine-particle air pollution on cold days. In New England, wood smoke is also a significant cause of air pollution—even worse than exhaust from car engines. And in Fort Collins, Colorado, wood smoke contributes to smog so severe it obscures visibility 1 out of 4 days.

If you burn wood for heat, make sure you do so in a stove that meets EPA standards. What about gas fireplaces that turn on with the flick of a switch? Many leak nitrogen dioxide and carbon monoxide into your home, so make sure they are fully vented to the outdoors.

Toss half-used cans of paint. Even when they're resealed, the paint can release significant levels of harmful VOCs. Unopened cans are more airtight but still emit fumes, so store them in a well-ventilated area, such as outdoors in a shed, until ready to use.

$10 AND UNDER

Lay off the fragrances. America's mania for pleasant scents (in the air and on our bodies) is making indoor air worse. Joint research from the Environmental Working Group and the University of Washington found that all top-selling laundry products emit at least one substance regulated as toxic or hazardous. And many air fresheners contain phthalates, hormone-disrupting chemicals that might affect reproductive development. It's best to choose soaps and cleaners free of perfumes and dyes. To scent your home, boil citrus peels or herbs like sage, rosemary, or mint.

Test for radon. Even though it's 100 percent natural, radon—an odorless, colorless, and tasteless radioactive gas found in one in 15 homes—is responsible for more than 21,000 lung cancer deaths each year. Home test kits cost as little at $10. (If you do have high levels of radon, the average cost of a mitigation system is $1,200.)

$30 AND UNDER

Make your own cleaners. Vinegar, borax, and baking soda can be used to clean your home without VOCs, says Dr. Sneller. Mix vinegar with water in a squirt bottle to spray down and wipe countertops; use baking soda in place of scouring powders and borax in toilets. Although strict environmentalists frown at the use of bleach as a disinfectant, public-health experts swear by its cost-effective ability to reduce mold. Use a simple solution of no more than 1 cup of bleach per 1 gallon of water. Just make sure to open the windows or run a fan while using it because the fumes can be irritating.

Buy a ficus plant. Researchers especially like them for their gas-absorbing and antimicrobial activity. They can even remove formaldehyde, one of the most potent VOCs released from some carpets and curtains, from the air. One study found that weeping fig and *Fatsia japonica* also efficiently remove formaldehyde from the air; another showed that purple heart and red and English ivies eliminate VOCs, like those off-gassed by paint. While more research is needed, start now to improve your air quality—one pot at a time.

Test your home's humidity levels. A simple way is to pick up a hygrometer from a local hardware store. Humidity levels should be between 30 and 60 percent, says Burton. Any higher levels might put you at risk for increases in mold and dust mites. (You should also consider purchasing a dehumidifier—good ones cost around $300.) Lower humidity levels can aggravate existing breathing problems and dry out your skin, so you may need a get a humidifier for your home. (They sell for around $120.)

journal

"MY FAMILY HELPED ME GET HEALTHY"

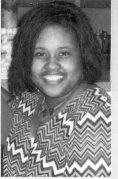

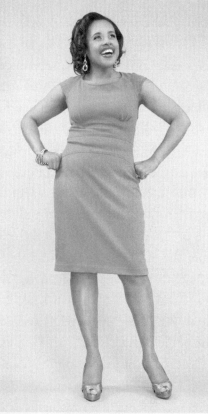

I leaned on my loved ones and got serious weight-loss results— 72 pounds, to be exact

by Tanzy Kilcrease

At the age of 30, I became the principal of an elementary school and went back to graduate school—all while raising my three children. I was too busy to cook, so we ate out for every meal. When I was stressed, I grabbed any sweet I could find. Soon the scale edged upward. I enrolled in diet and exercise programs, but nothing stuck. Instead of slimming down, I gained 70 pounds in 6½ years.

On January 1, 2007, my mother, aunt, and I were sitting around talking about how fat and tired we all were, and I couldn't stand it anymore. I said: "We can beat this. Let's start a group. We'll meet once a week, weigh in, and talk about what we've done to be healthy."

We started convening every Sunday at my mother's house. It was like our own private Weight Watchers meeting. We'd each get on the scale, then discuss strategies to help us meet our goals: Write in a journal to track food intake, increase our fiber by adding beans to our salads, or snack on fruit instead of chocolate to satisfy a sweet tooth. It was such great motivation. We screamed and gave each other high fives when we met our exercise or weight-loss goals for the week.

I lost 40 pounds the first 6 months. By the time I returned to school in the fall, I'd shed 55 pounds. My students didn't even recognize me! I've maintained my weight for more than 2 years, and people stop me all the time to ask how I did it. My answer: I'm still doing it. Losing weight and staying healthy is a lifelong journey.

Here are my top tips.

RISE AND SHINE. I squeeze in a 3-mile walk before work. It's the only time of day when I don't have appointments or social obligations to distract me.

GET TECH SAVVY. Online calorie trackers let you look up foods and keep tabs on daily intake with minimal calculations on your part. For a similar tool, go to www.prevention.com/myhealthtracker.

FIND A FRIEND. My neighbors are my walking buddies. I look forward to their company each morning, which means I'm more likely to stick with it.

MAKE ROOM FOR SPLURGES. I was a sugar addict, so I chose to give up daily processed sugar like candy, cookies, soda, and baked goods. But I still eat dessert on birthdays and special occasions so I don't feel deprived.

CLEAN OUT YOUR CLOSET. When I dropped a size, I donated everything in my closet that was too big. I didn't want any excuse to gain weight.

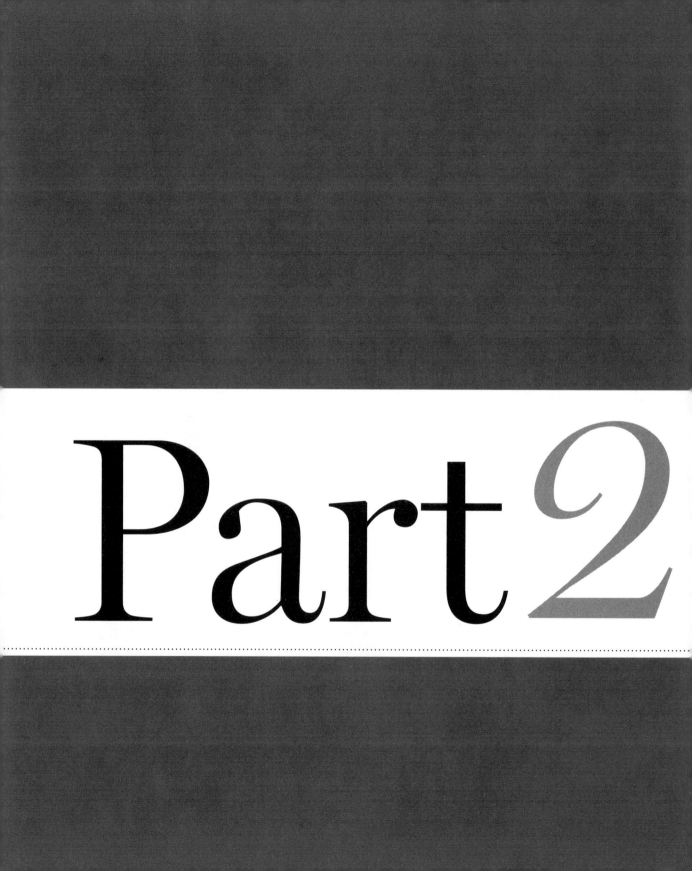

Part 2

WEIGHT-LOSS
WISDOM

CHAPTER 7

Eat Anything! Anywhere! Your 400 Calorie Fix

The only rule you need for permanent weight loss? Eat four 400-calorie meals a day. Slim has never been so simple!

The best formula for weight loss: Control your calories. You know it, we know it—and study after study proves it. So why is it that even though most of us aren't bingeing on high-fat fare or continually snacking on sweets, we're still gaining weight?

One reason is that 85 percent of adults have no idea how many calories they should consume to maintain a healthy weight. The other reason is that most of us don't know how many calories are in the foods we eat, and we don't have time to count them.

That's why *Prevention* created the new 400 Calorie Fix—a weight-loss plan that teaches you to control calories by limiting your meals to about 400 calories each.

"That's the right amount to allow for healthy variety in your diet and to keep you satisfied," explains nutritionist Mindy Hermann, RD, who helped create the plan. (To see how many 400-calorie meals you need daily, see Get Started Today, opposite page.)

How do you cap your meals without crunching numbers? By learning what 400 calories looks like. To help, we put together dozens of 400-calorie options, plus tips to control portions and spot hidden calories. You'll learn to see food through a 400-calorie lens whether you create meals at home or eat out.

What's more, we know it works: Sixteen women and men followed the plan and lost up to 11 pounds and 3 belly inches in just 2 weeks—and continued to lose in the months that followed.

Here are some simple ways to get started.

LEARN TO EYEBALL PORTION

When researchers asked study participants to estimate calories in restaurant entrees, they were off by as much as 100 percent. To estimate how many calories are in any given meal, you need to know how much food is on your plate. At home, you can weigh and measure with cups and scales, but when dining out, use these tricks to consume healthy portions:

- Thumb tip or 1 small marble = 1 teaspoon (for example, oil or jam)
- Thumb tip to first knuckle or 1 large marble = 1 tablespoon (for example, peanut butter)
- Thumb or 2 large marbles = 2 tablespoons solid food (for example, nuts) or 1 ounce liquid (for example, salad dressing)
- Golf ball or cupped handful = $\frac{1}{4}$ cup (for example, beans)
- Hockey puck or palm = 3 ounces (for example, cooked meat, poultry, or fish)
- Tennis ball = $\frac{1}{2}$ cup (for example, fruit)
- Your fist or a baseball = 1 cup (for example, vegetables or pasta)

SPOT HIDDEN FAT AND SUGAR

They can sneak into your meals and load them with unexpected calories. When you're doing the cooking, just swap in low-fat ingredients, such as reduced-fat salad dressings, cheese, and milk.

Dining out can be trickier. Watch for these signs your food is soaked in fat: pools of oil on the plate, a high-gloss shine or white coating on foods that aren't naturally white, or a dark stain or oil ring on a paper bag or plate. Finally, know that sugar is plentiful in soft drinks, desserts, and candy—and in foods you might not expect, such as ketchup and crackers. Read labels to spot hidden sugar sources (such as high fructose corn syrup and dextrose) or choose sugar-free alternatives.

SPLIT YOUR PLATE SIX WAYS

Sure, you can polish off 400 calories of chocolate cake and call it a meal, but you'll stay satisfied longer and eat healthier if you consume the right mix of veggies, fruits, proteins, and grains. For balanced nutrition and no-brainer calorie control, divide your plate into six equal sections: Fill one section with protein, two with grain, and the remaining three with fruits and veggies. This trick won't apply to every meal, but use it as a handy guide to eat in a way that boosts health and energy.

GET STARTED TODAY

On the pages that follow, you'll find nearly 50 meals that deliver between 370 and 420 calories each—from delicious recipes and quick no-cook meals you can make at home to options you can choose from when dining out, including takeout, Chinese and Italian restaurants, buffets, and even fast food. We did all the calorie counting for you. All you have to do is mix and match the meals you and your family like most and that fit your lifestyle best for a total of three, four, or five meals a day, depending on your personal weight-loss goal and activity level.

To jump-start your weight loss: If you're sedentary or moderately active, eat three 400-calorie meals a day for a combined 1,200 daily calories. Do this for 2 weeks and you can lose up to 11 pounds! (If you're very active and work out more than 60 minutes a day, choose four meals.)

To reach and maintain a healthy weight: Eat four 400-calorie meals a day for a combined 1,600 daily calories (perfect for a woman of average size who has an average activity level to achieve and stay at an ideal body weight). If you're very active, choose five meals.

400-CALORIE BUFFET

Heading to a restaurant featuring a buffet of foods—meats, fish, veggies, side dishes and more? Nothing is off-limits: This guide to healthy portions keeps calories in check. But if you stick to lean meats and veggies, you can even go back for seconds.

Roast Turkey: 2 slices roast turkey breast; 1 tablespoon turkey gravy

90 calories

Turkey breast is the leanest meat choice.

Baked Haddock: 4 ounces baked haddock; 1 tablespoon lemon-butter sauce

230 calories

Skip the sauce, and it's half the calories.

Roast Ham: 3-ounce slice

210 calories

Watch portions. It's fattier than ham from the deli.

Flank Steak: 3-ounce slice

170 calories

Drain off sauce when you scoop it to save calories.

Fried Chicken: 1 breast

360 calories

Fried Chicken: 1 drumstick

190 calories

The skin, batter, and frying oil equal high calories.

Rice Pilaf: 1 cup

230 calories

Oil and other ingredients make it higher in calories than plain white or brown rice.

Small Roll

90 calories

A small roll weighs about an ounce and should fit in your cupped hand.

Glazed Carrots: ½ cup

110 calories

The glaze adds 80 calories to an otherwise low-calorie option.

Roasted Potatoes: ½ cup

90 calories

Calories will be higher if the potatoes are shiny or sitting in a pool of oil.

Green Beans Amandine: ½ cup

90 calories

Calories are estimated based on 1 teaspoon each oil and almonds per serving. If it's shiny and drenched in sauce, amounts could be higher.

Smart 400-Calorie Combos

At the buffet, here are some terrific, yet still low-cal, pairings.

2 slices turkey + 1 tablespoon gravy + ¾ cup green beans amandine + ½ cup roasted potatoes + 1 small dinner roll = 405 calories

4 ounces baked haddock + 1 tablespoon lemon-butter sauce + ¼ cup glazed carrots + ½ cup rice pilaf = 400 calories

400-CALORIE ITALIAN

The challenge with this cuisine is portion size. In Italy, the pasta course is about appetizer size; in the United States, it's big enough to feed Mom, Dad, and all the kids. Here are tips to keep servings and calories in check.

Meat Lasagna: 10 ounces

420 calories

One serving is the size of fist plus a golf ball.

Penne alla Vodka: 1 cup penne + ½ cup vodka sauce

350 calories

Fried Calamari: about 1½ cups

400 calories

Spaghetti and Meatballs: 1 cup spaghetti + two 1-ounce meatballs + ½ cup tomato sauce

410 calories

Veal Marsala: 5 ounces

390 calories

Veal is the size of a hockey puck, and the mushrooms together would be the size of a golf ball.

Mozzarella Sticks: 4 sticks + 6 tablespoons marinara sauce
 390 calories

Fast Fixes

Here are some simple ways to cut back on calories while eating Italian.

- Ask for half-size portions of your main dish if possible, or split an entrée with a friend.
- Eyeball proper servings. For pasta, it's about the size of a baseball; for protein, the size of a hockey puck.
- Order extra vegetables. Salad with a little oil and vinegar is better than sautéed vegetables, however, which are often prepared with too much oil.
- Choose plain tomato or red clam sauce most often. They contain less fat and calories than other types. One-half cup of red sauce, for example, has about one-third the calories of Alfredo.

400-CALORIE CHINESE

Order your favorite items, then use our strategies to mix and match to create a 400-calorie plate. Bonus: You'll take home tomorrow's lunch as leftovers.

Steamed Vegetable Dumplings: 2 pieces
 110 calories

General Tso's Chicken: ½ cup
 290 calories

Hot and Sour Soup: 1 cup
 80 calories

Kung Pao Shrimp: ½ cup
 130 calories

White Rice: ½ cup
 100 calories

Smart 400-Calorie Combos

At the Chinese restaurant, here are some terrific, yet still low-cal, pairings.

1 cup soup + 2 dumplings + ½ cup white rice + ½ cup Kung Pao shrimp = 420 calories

2 dumplings + ½ cup General Tso's Chicken = 400 calories

Fast Fixes

Here are some simple ways to cut back on calories while eating Chinese.

- Start with a cup of broth-based soup or steamed dumplings. They're relatively low in calories and can help tame your appetite.
- Limit white or brown rice to ½ cup. Here's a neat trick: Use the Chinese tea cups on your table as portion guide; one holds about half a cup. Fried rice has up to twice the calories of plain and should be considered an entrée.
- Ask for sauce on the side, and use very little. Brown, sweet and sour, hoisin, and duck or plum sauce contain up to 5 teaspoons of sugar per ¼ cup.

400-CALORIE DRIVE-THRU

We all know fast food can be fattening, but close to half of us love it too much to give it up. Here's how to keep calories on track.

Burger King Small Fries:

340 calories

McDonald's Small Fries:

230 calories

Wendy's Sour Cream and Chives Baked Potato:

320 calories

Burger King Medium Onion Rings:

400 calories

McDonald's Quarter Pounder:

410 calories

Burger King Double Hamburger:

360 calories

McDonald's Filet-O-Fish Sandwich:

380 calories

Burger King BK Big Fish Sandwich (without tartar sauce):

460 calories

Wendy's Premium Fish Fillet Sandwich (without tartar sauce):

390 calories

McDonald's McChicken Sandwich:

360 calories

Wendy's Crispy Chicken Sandwich:

360 calories

Burger King Chicken Tenders (8 pieces):

360 calories

McDonald's Chicken McNuggets (7 pieces):

320 calories

With 1 package BBQ sauce:

370 calories

Fast Fixes

Here are some simple ways to cut back on calories while at the drive-thru.

- Say no to value deals that add extra items, and, when possible, split a meal with a friend so you can have a burger and the fries.
- Be picky. Ask for no mayonnaise. At about 100 calories per tablespoon, mayo (and sauces made with it, such as tartar sauce and ranch dressing) can add up to almost half your calories for the meal.
- Bulk up your meal by adding calorie-safe vegetable toppings such as lettuce, tomato, pickles, and sliced onions.
- Look up calorie counts at your favorite chain, because portion sizes can vary. A small order of fries at McDonald's, for example, has 110 fewer calories than the small size at Burger King.

400-CALORIE PARTY

A party can be a scary setting for a dieter, but if you choose wisely, you can enjoy your favorite treat and still stay within 400 calories.

Crudités: 1 cup

50 calories

Have a serving the size of your fist.

Pigs in a Blanket: 5 pigs

350 calories

Chex Mix: 1 cup

200 calories

A serving is the size of your fist.

Mini Chicken Satay Skewers: 2 skewers

60 calories

Mini Mushroom Turnovers: 2

80 calories

Pumpkin Pie: 1 slice

320 calories

One slice of pie is about half the size of your hand.

Apple Pie: 1 slice

410 calories

Caesar Salad: ½ cup

75 calories

A half cup of salad is the size of a tennis ball.

Tortellini Salad: ½ cup

190 calories

Sugar Cookies: 2

100 calories

Choose cookies that are each about the diameter of a golf ball.

Chocolate Chip Cookies: 2

120 calories

Soft Goat Cheese: 1 ounce

80 calories

One ounce of cheese is the size of your thumb or 2 large marbles.

Brie: 1 ounce
  100 calories
Cheddar Cheese: 1 ounce
  110 calories
Wine: 5-ounce glass
  125 calories
Champagne: 5-ounce glass
  110 calories

Smart 400-Calorie Combos

At a party, here are some delicious pairings that won't break the calorie bank.

5 ounces champagne + 1 cup crudités + 2 mini mushroom turnovers + 1 cup Caesar salad = 390 calories

1 cup Chex Mix + 1 ounce Cheddar cheese + 2 chocolate chip cookies = 430 calories

400-CALORIE RECIPES

From pancakes to chicken and pesto sandwiches, each of these recipes contains between 370 and 420 calories and is satisfying and easy to make. Choose three, four, or five meals a day, based on your weight-loss goals and activity level.

Breakfast

Hot Cereal: Bring 1 cup low-fat or fat-free milk to a boil, then add ¼ cup grain cereal (such as Bob's Red Mill 7 Grain or 10 Grain). Cover, simmer, and cook for 10 minutes, stirring occasionally. Top with 2 tablespoons pecans and ¼ cup dried apricot halves. Total: 380 calories

Bagel Egg Sandwich: Scoop out a 4" whole wheat bagel. Fill with 1 sliced hard-cooked egg, 1 tablespoon Miracle Whip Light, 2 tomato slices, and 2 lettuce leaves. Serve with a large coffee and 3 ounces low-fat milk. Total: 410 calories

Smoothie: Blend together 1 cup low-fat or fat-free milk, ¼ cup old-fashioned oats, 1 small banana, ½ cup berries, and 1 tablespoon peanut butter. Total: 390 calories

Cornmeal Pancakes: In a bowl, combine ½ cup cornmeal, ½ cup flour, ½ tablespoon baking powder, and ¼ teaspoon salt. Add ¾ cup low-fat or fat-free milk, 1 large egg, 2 tablespoons vegetable oil, 2 tablespoons honey, and ½ teaspoon vanilla extract. Stir well.

Heat a large skillet over medium heat and coat with cooking spray. Ladle about ¼ cup of the batter to make 4" pancakes. Cook until the bubbles on top have popped and the pancake appears firm but not dry. Flip and cook until the underside is done. (Makes 8 pancakes; 1 serving = 2 pancakes.) Total: 240 calories per serving

Raisin Bran Muffin: Choose a 2-ounce raisin bran muffin (about the size of a standard cupcake). Cut it in half and spread 1 teaspoon all-fruit strawberry jam on both sides. Serve with ¾ cup low-fat plain yogurt mixed with 1 cup fresh or frozen berries and 1 tablespoon wheat germ. Total: 420 calories

Lunch

Veggie Pizza: Preheat the oven to 450°F and place 1 package (15 to 16 ounce) refrigerated whole wheat pizza dough on the counter.

In a large skillet, heat 1 tablespoon olive oil. Add 1 cup sliced mushrooms and 1 cup sliced onions and stir briefly. Cover the pan and cook for 3 minutes. Remove the cover and cook for 5 minutes longer, or until almost all of the liquid boils off. Add ¼ teaspoon sea salt and remove from the heat.

Form the pizza dough into a ball and roll it out on a large, lightly floured baking sheet until it measures no thicker than ¼". Spread ½ cup pasta sauce on the dough and sprinkle with 1 cup grated part-skim mozzarella and ¼ cup grated Parmesan cheese. Top with the mushrooms and onions.

Bake for 25 minutes, or until the crust is lightly browned and the cheese is bubbly. (Cut into 8 slices; 1 serving = 2 slices.) Total: 400 calories per serving

Chef's Salad: Combine 2 cups mixed greens with a 1-ounce slice each turkey, ham, and roast beef, cut into thin strips; 5 sliced olives; 1 tomato, diced; ½ green bell pepper, diced; and 1 tablespoon sliced almonds. Toss with 1 tablespoon balsamic vinegar and 1 teaspoon olive oil. For dessert, have ½ cup low-fat frozen yogurt. Total: 410 calories

Macaroni Tuna Melt: In a microwave- or oven-safe bowl, mix together

⅔ cup cooked macaroni, ½ cup rinsed and drained light tuna, ¼ cup grated reduced-fat Cheddar cheese, 1 diced tomato, 2 tablespoons minced red onion, and 1 tablespoon Miracle Whip Light. Cook until heated through. Total: 390 calories

Grilled Chicken and Pesto Sandwich: Put 3 ounces grilled chicken (about the size of a hockey puck), 2 tomato slices, and 1 tablespoon pesto between 2 slices of whole grain bread. Serve with 1 cup broccoli florets drizzled with 1 tablespoon fat-free ranch dressing. Total: 410 calories

Dinner

Spicy Black Bean Soup and Tortillas: Soak 1½ cups dried black beans overnight. The next morning, drain the beans and place them in a slow cooker with 5 cups water, 1 cup chopped yellow onion, ½ pound chopped red potatoes, 1 cup salsa, and 2 cloves minced garlic. Cover and cook on low for 8 hours, or until the beans are soft.

Season with ½ teaspoon sea salt and ⅛ teaspoon ground black pepper. Top with 6 tablespoons shredded four-cheese blend, 6 tablespoons low-fat plain yogurt, and 6 tablespoons minced cilantro. (1 serving = 1½ cups.) Total: 240 calories per serving

Pair with 2 warmed tortillas and a small green salad for a combined 390 calories.

Shrimp Teriyaki Noodle Bowl: Toss 1 cup cooked whole wheat spaghetti with 4 ounces frozen shrimp (thawed and cooked per package directions), 1 cup frozen broccoli (cooked per package directions), and 2 tablespoons low-sodium teriyaki sauce. Top with ¼ cup water chestnuts. Total: 390 calories

Sweet and Tangy Mustard-Molasses Chicken: Preheat the oven to 400°F. Remove the skin from 2 pounds bone-in chicken breasts and place in a pan. (If the chicken breasts are large—about 1 pound each—cut them in half.) Top with 1 thinly sliced onion.

Combine ¼ cup deli mustard and ¼ cup molasses and brush onto the chicken breasts. Bake for 25 minutes, or until cooked through, turning the chicken halfway through. (Makes 4 servings; 1 serving = ¼ pound chicken breast.) Total: 280 calories per serving

Serve with oven-baked fries: Cut half a potato into wedges, toss with ½ teaspoon olive oil and salt-free seasoning, and bake for 20 to 30 minutes, until crisp, for a combined 380 calories.

Vegetable Medley Salad: Combine 2 cups romaine or mixed lettuce; ½ cup rinsed and drained canned chickpeas; 1 slice Alpine Lace Swiss cheese, cut into strips; 1 tomato, cut into wedges; ¼ cup sliced cucumber; and ½ cup plain croutons. Toss with a few shakes of salt-free seasoning, 2 teaspoons olive oil, and 1 tablespoon balsamic vinegar. Total: 400 calories

Grilled Salmon: Prepare 1 frozen salmon fillet (such as Gorton's Classic Grilled Salmon) according to package directions. Serve with ½ cup whole grain brown rice and 1 cup cooked mixed vegetables (such as Green Giant's Simply Steam Broccoli & Carrots). Enjoy with 4 gingersnap cookies. Total: 410 calories

Snacks

Cookies and Milk: Dip five Oreos in 1 cup low-fat or fat-free milk. Total: 370 calories

Frozen Yogurt Pie: Preheat the oven to 350°F. Grind 20 graham cracker squares into crumbs (makes about 1 cup). Reserve 1 tablespoon crumbs and combine the rest with 3 tablespoons melted unsalted butter. Pat firmly into an 8" pie pan and bake for 10 minutes, then cool completely.

Gently fold two 6-ounce cartons blended raspberry yogurt into 2 cups Cool Whip Lite. Spoon into the pie dish, cover, and freeze until firm (at least 3 hours).

Remove the pie from the freezer 30 minutes before serving. Top with 2 cups thawed frozen raspberries before cutting. (Makes 8 servings; 1 serving = 1 of 8 wedges.) Total: 210 calories per serving

Enjoy with latte made with ¾ cup low-fat milk and 3 blocks Hershey's Special Dark chocolate for a combined 400 calories.

Molten Brownie Bites: Preheat the oven to 400°F. Coat a 24-cup mini muffin pan with cooking spray.

Pour one 17- to 20-ounce box Ghirardelli Chocolate Brownie Mix into a large bowl. In a smaller bowl, beat 2 eggs, 1 egg yolk, and ¼ cup low-fat mayonnaise with an electric mixer on high speed for about 2 minutes. Add to the brownie mix, along with $\frac{1}{2}$ cup melted unsalted butter.

Spoon the batter into the muffin pan, filling each cup to the top. Bake for 10 minutes, then immediately remove the bites from the pan with a tablespoon. (Makes 12 servings; 1 serving = 2 brownie bites.) Total: 300 calories per serving

Enjoy with 1 cup low-fat or fat-free milk for a combined 400 calories.

Chips and Guacamole: Mash $\frac{1}{4}$ cup avocado with $\frac{1}{4}$ cup salsa. Serve with 2 ounces tortilla chips (about 20 chips). Total: 400 calories

400-CALORIE GIRLS' NIGHT OUT

Yes, you can live it up with your friends and still keep your meal around 400 calories. That's the right amount to help you lose weight and stay satisfied (margaritas included).

Out for Mexican: Order regular-size nachos for the table (about one-quarter of the plate is 205 calories) and a small frozen margarita for yourself (190 calories in 6 ounces)—the added ice helps dilute the drink and stretch the calories. If the bar uses real fruit, ask for a strawberry margarita instead of plain (for an extra dose of vitamins). Total: 395 calories

In your living room: Serve soft cheese, which has fewer calories than hard (1 thumb-size ounce of goat cheese is 75 calories); 2 rye crispbreads (75 calories); apple slices (half a small apple has 40 calories); and dark chocolate (2 blocks of Hershey's Special Dark have 75 calories). Enjoy with a 5-ounce glass of red wine (125 calories). Total: 390 calories

Happy hour: Snack on some tiny twist pretzels first ($\frac{1}{2}$ ounce, or about half a Wiffle ball's worth, is 50 calories); they'll help absorb the alcohol. Then enjoy a 3-ounce martini (170 calories) and a 5-ounce glass of white wine (120 calories) while noshing on two chicken satay skewers (60 calories). Total: 400 calories

Pizza night: Order a thin-crust slice (to cut down on carb calories), but top it with peppers, broccoli, and mushrooms to make it more filling (260 calories). Or split a personal-size veggie pie with a friend (half is about 275 calories). Pair either one with a bottle of beer for 150 calories. Total: 410 to 425 calories

400-CALORIE SALAD BAR

Use this portion guide to build a hunger-busting salad and keep calories in check. Aim for about 400 calories total—the right amount per meal to help you lose weight and stay satisfied.

Greens: 1 cup (baseball size)

10 calories

Darker leaves pack more nutrients, so choose mixed greens over iceberg lettuce.

Chickpeas or kidney beans: ¼ cup (golf ball size)

70–90 calories

Mixed beans in a dressing contain extra fat, so drain the liquid.

Chopped egg: 2 tablespoons (or 2 large marbles)

30 calories

Eat just the egg white and you'll save half the calories.

Tomatoes: ½ cup (tennis ball size)

20 calories

If they're shiny, they've been tossed in oil, which means more calories.

Sliced ham or turkey: 2 tablespoons

30 calories

Both are high in protein and low in fat; if the ham is cut into chunks, however, it may not be as lean.

Avocado: ¼ cup

60 calories

Though high in calories, it's rich in good fats, which can help you feel full.

Shredded cheese: 2 tablespoons

60 calories

Assume that all the cheeses are full-fat.

Cucumbers: ¼ cup

5 calories

They're so low in calories, feel free to pile them high.

Fat-free dressing: 2 tablespoons

20–50 calories

Light dressing: 2 tablespoons

50–80 calories

Regular dressing: 2 tablespoons

100–150 calories

Vinaigrettes tend to have fewer calories than creamy ones.

Smart 400-Calorie Combo

When you're at a salad bar, choose this combo for just a pinch over 400 calories.

2 cups mixed greens + 1 cup sliced cucumbers + 1 cup tomatoes + ½ cup chickpeas + 2 tablespoons regular dressing = 410 calories

400-CALORIE BALLGAME

Ballpark classics aren't exactly health food, but if you pay attention to portions, you can still keep your stadium meal or snack to around 400 calories—the right amount to help you lose weight and stay satisfied.

Hot Dog and Seltzer: Get a quarter-pound hot dog with bun (400 calories) or a large corn dog (380 calories) and top with two small-marble-size squirts of mustard (5 calories). Add seltzer and you're set. Sprinkle on a tablespoon of onion (5 calories for the size of a large marble) for a flavor boost. Total: 390 to 410 calories

Chicken Tenders and Onion Rings: Split an order of chicken tenders with a friend. Three pieces dipped in 2 tablespoons barbecue sauce is 190 calories. Pair with onion rings (seven for 215 calories). For a dose of potassium, substitute 30 to 35 small fries (2.5 ounces, 225 calories) for the onion rings. Total: 405 to 415 calories

Nachos and Beer: If the chips are thin, eat nine for 130 calories; if thick, nosh on five. Dip in 2 ounces—four large marbles—of cheese (120 calories), and enjoy a 12-ounce beer (150 calories). Add a few tablespoons of jalapeño peppers for more than 10 percent of daily vitamins A and C. Total: 400 calories

Nuts and Candy: Peanuts are packed with calories (1,200 per bag at Yankee Stadium!). Stick to ⅔ cup, just bigger than a tennis ball (230 calories). Add 1½ ounces cotton candy (a softball) for 150 calories. Share your snacks to keep portions in check. Total: 380 calories

CHAPTER 8

Busted! Hidden Diet Disasters

Thanks to confusing labels and unearned reputations, it's difficult to know what's good for you these days. From veggie chips to Greek yogurt, here are "healthy" foods that really aren't

If you're reading this book (and the evidence is pretty good that you are), you're probably interested in buying the healthiest foods. Just like us, you may even reach automatically for items with a "health halo," such as spaghetti sauce (love that lycopene!), or labels like *reduced fat!, low sodium!,* and *whole grain!* But unless you're a supersavvy shopper, be warned: Your diet may conceal some nasty surprises.

That low-fat cottage cheese you love? It could be higher in sodium than potato chips. And the low-fat dressing you drizzle on your salad? It could contain nearly as much sugar as two chocolate chip cookies.

The truth is that no manufacturer wants to compromise on flavor, so even healthy-sounding products can contain appalling levels of sugar, salt, and bad fats. To save you time, we've flushed out some of the most surprising offenders—and found some truly healthful alternatives.

DISASTER: SNEAKY SALT

Even foods that sound healthy can be loaded with salt, and that can spell trouble. Most Americans already consume double the daily recommended amount of sodium—currently set at 1,500 milligrams, or about ⅔ teaspoon of table salt. (The limit was just lowered by the National Academy of Sciences and the American Heart Association from 2,300 milligrams a day.)

If you're in the high-intake group, that could significantly escalate your blood pressure and increase your risk of strokes and heart attacks—even if your blood pressure is normal, says Elisa Zied, RD, author of *Nutrition at Your Fingertips.*

CULPRIT: McDonald's Premium Caesar Salad with Grilled Chicken contains 890 milligrams of sodium—more than half the recommended daily limit. And that's without the Caesar dressing, which can pile on another 500 milligrams. (Select the low-fat Italian and it's even 30 percent higher!)

In these ready-to-go salads, says Lona Sandon, RD, an assistant professor of clinical nutrition at the University of Texas Southwestern Medical Center, "the worst part is usually the chicken, which is often cooked in a high-sodium

ARE BOTTLED TEAS A BUST?

You'd likely never drink 20 bottles of tea in a day, but that's how much you would have to sip of some brands to get the same amount of disease-fighting polyphenols as 1 cup of brewed tea. In a 2010 study, researchers analyzed 49 brands of bottled tea and found that most had very low or no antioxidants. What they did have was plenty of sugar. So stick to tea bags, and if it's iced tea you want, brew your own and chill it right away to help preserve more antioxidants, says Shiming Li, PhD, lead author of the study. If you must add sweetener, go easy.

20

THE PERCENTAGE REDUCTION IN CALORIES
EATEN IN YOUR MAIN COURSE WHEN YOU HAVE
SOUP FIRST, ACCORDING TO THE PENNSYLVANIA
STATE UNIVERSITY

marinade for flavor and may also be injected with a sodium solution to keep the meat moist."

Smarter choice: Skip the entrée salad and go for the burger with a garden salad on the side. A McDonald's plain hamburger has 520 milligrams of sodium (250 calories, 9 grams fat); add the side salad (20 calories, 0 grams fat, 10 milligrams sodium) or snack-size fruit-and-walnut salad (210 calories, 8 grams fat, 60 milligrams sodium).

CULPRIT: Bertolli Roasted Chicken & Linguine packs a whopping 1,350 milligrams of sodium in a serving. And if you eat both servings in the 24-ounce package (it's not a stretch), you'll consume almost double your daily sodium in one sitting. Like other manufacturers, Bertolli uses the preservative sodium phosphate in addition to table salt to flavor this frozen entrée.

Smarter choice: Amy's Kitchen Light in Sodium Black Bean Enchilada has just 190 milligrams of sodium per serving.

CULPRIT: Near East Spanish Rice Pilaf contains 910 milligrams of sodium in its 2.5-ounce serving (240 calories, 0.5 gram fat)—nearly two-thirds of the recommended daily dose (and more if you add butter as suggested). That's high, even by the standards of these supersimple dishes, which generally contain about 500 to 800 milligrams of sodium.

Smarter choice: Near East Original Plain Whole Grain Wheat Couscous contains no salt; simply season with your own spice blend. Bonus: Many herbs and spices like cilantro and turmeric are packed with disease-fighting phytonutrients.

CULPRIT: Breakstone's Fat-Free Cottage Cheese has 400 milligrams of sodium per 4-ounce serving (70 calories). That's like eating 2¼ one-ounce bags of Lay's potato chips. In order to give cottage cheese its curds-and-whey consistency, manufacturers must add salt during production. This salt, plus the natural salt contained in the milk used to make the cheese, gives this typical health fixture a surprisingly high sodium level.

Smarter choice: Equally creamy and still diet friendly, Sorrento Low-Fat Ricotta (140 milligrams sodium and 100 calories per 4 ounces) is worth trying.

DISASTER: SNEAKY SUGAR

You know that treats such as soda, ice cream, and cookies are loaded with the sweet stuff. But various forms of sugar—especially high fructose corn syrup—sneak into a wide array of savory items, too, where you would hardly expect to find them.

"When you remove fat, you also remove moisture, so manufacturers add sugar to help retain moisture and flavor," notes Sandon. Besides the obvious danger to your teeth and your waistline, excess sugar ups your risk of heart disease. Remember: Your recommended limit is 25 grams of added sugar a day (about 6 teaspoons, or 100 calories).

CULPRIT: Prego Traditional Italian Sauce sounds so healthful. (How could "traditional" marinara be anything other than wholesome?) But its third ingredient is sugar, which is added to balance out the acidity. Combined with the natural sugars in the tomatoes, that makes for a total of 10 grams per serving.

Smarter choice: Muir Glen Organic Garlic Roasted Garlic Pasta Sauce has only 4 grams of sugar per serving. For an option that's also low salt, try Amy's Organic Light in Sodium Marinara Sauce (5 grams sugar and just 100 milligrams sodium).

CULPRIT: At 33 grams per 8-ounce glass, Ocean Spray Cranberry Juice Cocktail has as much sugar as a can of soda. (The word *cocktail* is a red flag.)

Smarter choice: For a refreshing (and guilt-free!) alternative, try flavored seltzer, such as Vintage Raspberry Seltzer (0 grams added sugar).

CULPRIT: Häagen-Dazs Lowfat Vanilla Frozen Yogurt has 21 grams of sugar in a half-cup serving—nearly double the amount in real ice cream such as Edy's Grand French Vanilla (11 grams) and close to your limit for the entire day.

Smarter choice: Edy's Whole Fruit No Sugar Added Fruit Bars will satisfy your sweet tooth with just 2 grams of sugar and only 30 calories per serving (0 grams fat).

CULPRIT: Maple Grove Farms Fat Free Honey Dijon Salad Dressing has 8 grams of sugar in 2 tablespoons. That's like tossing 10 jelly beans into your salad.

Smarter choice: Newman's Own Lighten Up Balsamic Vinaigrette has just 1 gram of sugar (and 4 grams fat). Wish-Bone Light Italian has 2 grams of sugar (2.5 grams fat).

DISASTER: SNEAKY FAT

If low-fat foods add sugar to make up for missing flavor, then full-fat varieties must be healthy and satisfying, right? Not when you look over labels with an expert eye. One pitfall is heart-stopping saturated and trans fats, which increase blood sugar levels, blunt insulin resistance, and decrease your ratio of good to bad cholesterol. Then there's the serving size, which can trick you into thinking you're getting a dollop of fat—when you are actually getting most of a day's serving. Overall, try to keep fats to 35 percent of caloric intake. (In a 1,600-calorie diet, that's 62 grams.)

CULPRIT: Calbee Snack Salad Snapea Crisps may be vegetable based—and baked—but they still have 8 grams of fat per 1-ounce serving. That's almost as much as a small bag of Lay's potato chips.

Smarter choice: For a chiplike feel with a protein bonus, try Glenny's Lightly Salted Soy Crisps, which have just 1 gram of fat per serving (5 grams protein and only 170 milligrams sodium). If you're looking for vegetables, try Just Tomatoes, Etc.! Just Veggies, a mix of freeze-dried carrots, corn, peas, peppers, and tomatoes that has 1 gram of fat (4 grams protein and just 40 milligrams sodium).

CULPRIT: Fage Total Plain Classic Greek Yogurt has 23 grams of fat (18 grams saturated) and 300 calories in 1 cup. That's not to say there aren't good reasons to buy this ultrathick and creamy yogurt. It's a great source of calcium (you'll get 25 percent of your Daily Value in a 1-cup serving) and

THINK OUTSIDE THE CAN

Canned fruits, vegetables, and soups seem so healthful—and so easy to buy, store, and use. But 92 percent of the cans tested in a recent study had harmful bisphenol A, so we asked *Prevention* editors and readers to try more than a dozen soups in cartons (the linings are BPA free) to find the best-tasting, healthiest ones. All four of our top picks have filling fiber and protein, minimal fat, and no added sugar. Because soups tend to be salty, watch your total sodium intake (daily limit: 1,500 milligrams). The tasty low-sodium pick topping our list makes it easy.

DR. MCDOUGALL'S LIGHT SODIUM LENTIL: *Prevention* testers didn't miss the salt in this delicious soup. The veggies provide 20 percent of vitamins A and C, and the lentils are packed with protein. Per serving: 100 calories, 6 g protein, 18 g carbohydrates, 7 g fiber, 0.5 g total fat, 0 g saturated fat, 290 mg sodium

KETTLE CUISINE CHICKEN SOUP WITH RICE NOODLES: This classic comes in a microwaveable bowl and is ready in about 5 minutes. There isn't much fiber, but the chicken's protein left testers satisfied. Per serving: 140 calories, 15 g protein, 12 g carbohydrates, 1 g fiber, 3 g total fat, 0.5 g saturated fat, 560 mg sodium

DR. MCDOUGALL'S BLACK BEAN: This hearty blend of black beans, vegetables, and organic brown rice kept testers full for hours. There's just the right amount of spice, and cilantro adds great flavor. Per serving: 120 calories, 6 g protein, 23 g carbohydrates, 5 g fiber, 1 g total fat, 0 g saturated fat, 460 mg sodium

KETTLE CUISINE THREE BEAN CHILI: If you like spicy foods, you'll love this thick chili. It's loaded with pinto, chili, and black beans, plus tomatoes, peppers, and onions, which boost the fiber count. Per serving: 220 calories, 11 g protein, 36 g carbohydrates, 13 g fiber, 3.5 g total fat, 1 g saturated fat, 450 mg sodium

---

protein (15 grams), plus it has those good-for-your-gut live active cultures. But the whole-milk variety has five times the fat content of the 2 percent fat version and twice the calories (300, versus 150 in the 2 percent product).

Smarter choice: Fage Total 0% Plain Greek Yogurt is made with fat-free milk so it still provides all the calcium and cultures, and it even has a power-packed 20 grams of protein, all with no fat and just 120 calories.

CULPRIT: When you survey the king-size choices at the concession stand, movie popcorn doesn't look so bad. But think again: According to the Center for Science in the Public Interest, Regal (the country's biggest movie theater chain) serves a medium-size popcorn with 60 grams of saturated fat (and 1,200 calories)—as much as five Burger King Whoppers. The problem: It's popped in artery-clogging oils, then topped with even more offending fats in the buttery topping.

"They don't call them tubs for nothing," says CSPI senior nutritionist Jayne Hurley, RD.

Smarter choice: BYO. Newman's Own 94% Fat Free Microwave Popcorn has just 1.5 grams of fat per serving, none of it saturated or trans fat. (Just don't get caught.)

CULPRIT: Aidells Smoked Chicken and Apple Sausage has 11 grams of fat (3.5 grams saturated) and 160 calories per link (and really, who eats just one link?). Many brands of poultry sausage have only slightly less fat than typical sweet Italian sausage (12 grams) because they're often stuffed with some of the fattiest parts of the chicken, including the skin and dark meat.

Smarter choice: Low-fat grilled chicken breast has only 3 grams of fat (and 140 calories) in 3 ounces.

CULPRIT: Amy's Indian Paneer Tikka has 19 grams of fat (and 320 calories) in a 9½-ounce serving. You'd think going meatless would be a healthy choice, but you can blame the cheese (made with whole milk), as well as the oil the dish is cooked in.

Smarter choice: You don't need to swear off Indian completely. Amy's Indian Mattar Tofu provides protein (12 grams) and also delivers fiber (5 grams) with just 8 grams of fat.

CHAPTER 9

Splash-Slim

Lose weight and feel great! It doesn't take endless laps to see fantastic results from water workouts!

Whether it's 70 degrees and sunny or 30 degrees and snowing, if you have access to a pool, there's no time like the present to submerge yourself in some refreshing H_2O. And while you're at it, you can burn calories and tone up all over—faster, in fact, than if you exercised in the air-conditioned sanctuary of your gym. Why? Water provides 12 to 15 times more resistance than air. So you can burn as many as $3\frac{1}{2}$ times more calories than if you walked at a moderate pace—and it's more refreshing! You don't even have to swim to get these results.

Here are 18 easy ways to get started, from solo moves you can do in a pool or at the beach to high-energy games for the whole family. You'll have more fun, stay cool, and shed pounds in no time.

IF YOU'RE HANGING OUT AT THE POOL, TRY . . .

Treading intervals: They burn twice the calories of regular treading. You'll slim down faster and firm up all over. In deep water, tread as hard as you can for 30 seconds. Then go easy or float on your back for 30 seconds. Fit in 30 bursts over your afternoon at the pool and you'll scorch nearly 300 calories.

Step pushups: Make getting strong a snap! You're lighter in water, so full pushups are easier while still being a super arm and shoulder toner, says Rob Shapiro, a 16-year veteran personal trainer in Brookline, Massachusetts. Start in plank position in the shallow end, your hands on the top pool step and your toes on the pool floor. Slowly bend your elbows to lower as far as you can without getting your face wet. Straighten your elbows and repeat. Work up to two or three slow sets of 15 reps.

Waist-deep lunges: Shape your thighs without straining your knees. Water makes high-impact jumps joint friendly. In waist-deep water, lunge with your right foot forward, right thigh parallel to the pool floor, left knee bent, hands on your hips. Quickly jump up, scissor your legs, and land with your left leg forward. Do 15 to 20 times.

The blender: This move firms legs from every angle. Water workouts provide 360 degrees of resistance, says Jay Cardiello, a certified strength and conditioning specialist in New York City. In waist-deep water, quickly swing your right leg forward. Pause, then pull it back against the current to the starting position. Next, swing your leg to the side, then back. Alternate legs for 10 to 15 cycles.

The helicopter: "Jog" in the water to burn fat fast. This move revs your heart rate to melt more calories, says Mary Sanders, PhD, a spokesperson for the American Council on Exercise and director of WaterFit Wave Aerobics. Squat in waist- to rib cage-deep water, then jump up and "jog" vigorously for a count of six. Repeat for 1 minute, then rest for 15 seconds. Do two more times.

AT THE BEACH, TRY . . .

Surf strolling: You'll blast up to 180 percent more calories than from walking on pavement. The combo of sand and water kicks your lower-body muscles into high gear. Researchers found that walking in thigh-deep waves yields the biggest burn, but even ankle-deep water will tone your legs.

Wave jumping: Do squats without realizing it. Head out into waist-deep water, crouch down, and jump over the waves as they come in. Try jumping backward or sideways, or scissoring your legs.

The ocean push-and-pull: Play a balance game to sculpt sexy abs. Simply staying upright as the waves hit works your abs and back to tone your torso. Try balancing on one foot to work more muscles. Or compete with your pals to see who can remain standing the longest. (Up the ante by facing the beach so the waves surprise you.)

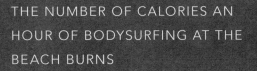

200
THE NUMBER OF CALORIES AN HOUR OF BODYSURFING AT THE BEACH BURNS

SMART PICKS AT THE SNACK BAR

You can keep calories in check even if the snack bar is your only dining option. Here are the top winners—and losers—of poolside eating, compliments of the *Eat This, Not That* book series.

IF YOU'RE CRAVING SALT, snack on a soft pretzel with mustard for only 290 calories.

PASS ON french fries, which pack a whopping 600 calories.

IF YOU WANT SOMETHING SWEET, snack on 10 SweeTarts for about 50 calories.

PASS ON Dots—11 pieces have 130 calories.

IF YOU'RE THIRSTY, sip on iced tea, just 4 calories.

PASS ON cola, which has about 150 calories a can.

IF YOU NEED A REAL MEAL, snack on a hot dog. Add relish, ketchup, and mustard and you'll consume only 320 calories.

PASS ON a cheeseburger. One 5-ounce burger has 630 calories.

FOR A DAY OF FAMILY FUN, TRY . . .

Chaos running: Splash off some calories. On the count of three, everyone carefully walks or jogs in a zigzag pattern from one end of the pool to the other, then back, suggests Dr. Sanders. The currents created by the erratic directions increase resistance.

Water circles: Massage your thighs in a do-it-yourself whirlpool. Walk as fast as you can in a circle around a section of the pool that's about 3 feet deep (the more people, the better the effect). Do about 20 laps, then change direction for 10 laps. The resulting rush of water against your body will feel much like the jets in a whirlpool.

A game of fetch: Torch 175 calories in just 20 minutes. Throw an inflatable ball to the other side of the pool and see who can retrieve it the fastest. You won't even notice you're doing sprints.

A trip to a water park: Boost your butt with a fun stair workout. You may climb more than 800 steps to reach the waterslides and walk 5 to 7 miles during a 1-day visit. And the ride down will cool you off.

IF THERE ARE FLOTATION TOOLS HANDY, TRY . . .

Kickboard laps: Target your fat-burning leg and butt muscles. You'll easily glide through the water with a kickboard or noodle in hand. Practice different types of kicking: flutter (alternating legs), dolphin (legs together, mermaid style), and breaststroke (frog kicks), suggests Paul Smith, swimming instructor and fitness specialist at Lake Austin Spa Resort in Austin, Texas.

Deepwater jogging: Burn a whopping 750 calories an hour. Hold a noodle or slip on a flotation belt or vest (available at most pools). "Run" as hard as you can for 30 to 60 seconds, bringing your knees toward your chest and pumping your arms. Do 10 sets, recovering your breath between sprints, suggests exercise physiologist and triathlon coach Ben Greenfield of Spokane, Washington.

A beach ball workout: Tone your arms and shoulders—no throwing (or catching) required. Trying to submerge a ball that floats really works your core and upper body. Experiment with different movements to vary the muscles targeted, says Dr. Sanders. For example, press a small ball down in front of you with bent arms, then move it to the side and straighten your arms.

IF YOU DON'T WANT TO GET YOUR HAIR WET, TRY . . .

Backward motion: Work more muscles for speedier results. Research shows that water walking or jogging in reverse engages more muscles in your legs and back than going forward (83 percent more quads, 61 percent more lower back, and 47 percent more calves).

Shuffle slides: Slim down saddlebags. To tone your inner and outer thighs, shuffle side to side in at least thigh-deep water, says Melissa Layne, an American Council on Exercise spokesperson and a water aerobics instructor for 20-plus years. Keep movements smooth.

Arm presses: Firm up as you chat—no one will notice! Stand in chest-deep water with your palms open and fingers spread and move your arms back and forth and up and down. Increase your speed for a greater challenge.

CHAPTER 10

The New Superslimmers

The results are in. Here's how switching up your strength routine with a new easy-to-use tool can transform your body in 3 short weeks!

You want to get strong and fit, but you don't have a lot of time to exercise. Enter kettlebells.

In just 20 minuses, these cannonball-shaped weights with a handle on top offer a workout that delivers more fat-fighting and body-toning benefits than doing 30 minutes on the treadmill and 30 minutes of traditional weight lifting, according to recent research from the American Council on Exercise.

This revved-up toning session features dynamic, multimuscle moves. Unlike typical strength exercises in which you lift and lower weights slowly while keeping the rest of your body still, you swing the kettlebell rhythmically through full-body motions to get your heart rate up fast and target

KETTLEBELL: ANATOMY OF A SUPERSLIMMER

Unlike a dumbbell, in which the weight is equally balanced when you hold it, a kettlebell is asymmetrical. With most grips, your hand is set away from the heaviest part of the kettle bell, so you work harder and activate more muscles.

HANDLE: Most common spot to hold, so you can swing the bell and pass it from hand to hand.

HORNS: Alternate grip, especially if you're holding the bell upside down.

BASE: The heaviest part of the bell. Gripping it here provides more stability.

more muscles, especially in your core. The result is a speedy routine that triples your calorie burn to up to 400 calories in 20 minutes.

What's more, our kettlebell-inspired routine (you can do it with a dumbbell, too), created by personal trainer and *Prevention* contributing editor Chris Freytag, was designed to produce maximum results with minimal risk of injury. And it delivered: When two dozen women road-tested it, they lost up to 11 pounds and 15 inches in just 3 weeks. Even better, they loved the workout!

"I heard the word *fun* used more than I ever had to describe a routine," says Freytag. "Getting in a rhythm with the swings and doing little tosses makes it less boring than just hoisting weights and gives you a little bit of that cardio high."

In addition to three kettlebell workouts a week, our test panel did 20 minutes of cardio on alternate days, and half of the group also followed a healthy eating plan.

Whether you have 20 or more pounds to lose, are struggling with those last stubborn 5, or want to firm up, now you can ring up results in just 20 minutes a day!

PROGRAM AT A GLANCE

What you'll need: A kettlebell, or you can substitute a dumbbell. Our testers used an 8.8-pound (4 kilogram) kettlebell ($29.95 at www.spri.com) and felt that it added to the fun and novelty of the routine. You'll also need a watch or timer, as well as space to swing your arms freely on all sides, including overhead (about 4 square feet).

Three days a week: Do the following kettlebell workout on nonconsecutive days. Do the Main Moves (see page 95) twice through for 16 minutes total. Then stretch for 2 minutes. Go to www.prevention.com/kettlestretch for cooldown ideas.

Three or 4 days a week: Do 20 minutes of cardio, such as brisk walking, lap swimming, jogging, dancing, or bike riding. You should exercise at an intensity at which you're breathing hard but can still speak in short sentences. Do cardio on the same day as kettlebells for longer workouts or on alternate days for shorter workouts.

Every day: Watch portions and fill up on whole grains, vegetables, fruits, lean protein, and healthy fats to maximize results. Aim for 1,600 to 1,800 calories spread evenly throughout the day. For help, go to www.prevention.com/portioncontrol.

KETTLEBELL: GROUND RULES

Follow these technique and form tips for safer toning.

STAND TALL. Keep shoulders back and down, chest lifted.

CONTRACT YOUR CORE. Before beginning each move, tighten your ab muscles as if someone threw very cold water on your belly. Maintain this contraction throughout the exercise, but don't hold your breath.

STAY IN CONTROL. Move rhythmically, but don't fling the weight.

WE LOVED IT!

"I was shocked to lose 11 pounds in just 3 weeks."—Gretchen Streete, 40

As a mother of three young children, Gretchen has little time to exercise and, despite trying a variety of workouts, was unable to find something she could stick with—until now. "Kettlebells don't take a lot of time," she says. "I did the routine while my kids played outside or watched TV." She also reports having more energy!

"I lost 3+ inches off my waist and 2+ from each thigh."—Cheryl Bechel, 43

This was the first time that Cheryl had ever done any type of strength training, and she loved it! The fast-paced, quick workout was just what this mother of two teenagers needed. Last year she lost 40 pounds, but 10 had crept back on. In just 3 weeks, she dropped 6½ of them—without dieting. "My clothes fit so well now," she says. And after 6 weeks, she was confidently swinging a 15-pound kettlebell. "That was encouraging," she adds.

"It's so easy to do!"—Beth Ulrich, 40

After losing and regaining the same 10 pounds over the past 5 years, Beth was looking for a workout that she could stick with to keep the pounds off for good. And she found it. "Kettlebells are so simple—just eight exercises and only 20 minutes," says this busy working mom, who lost 7 pounds in 4 weeks. "After just 2 weeks, I could zip up my pants without holding my breath."

"I'm stronger and more confident."—Lora Bloomquist, 42

As Lora prepares to fulfill a lifelong dream of opening her own vintage furniture shop, she knows it's time to refurbish her body as well. "I will be on my feet more, moving and lifting furniture," she explains. And she noticed the results almost immediately. "My muscles felt stronger," says the mother of three, who lost more than 10 pounds in 3 weeks. After 2 weeks, she reported that her jeans were looser, and at week 3, she noticed her arms looked firmer and smaller. "I feel great inside—and out."

Chris Freytag is a board member of the American Council on Exercise, star of many *Prevention* Fitness Systems DVDs, and author of *Prevention's 2-Week Total Body Turnaround.*

. . . .

WARMUP

(2 minutes) Stand with your feet hip-width apart for all three exercises. You can do these with a lighter kettlebell (or dumbbell) or no weight at all if you want to ease into the workout more slowly.

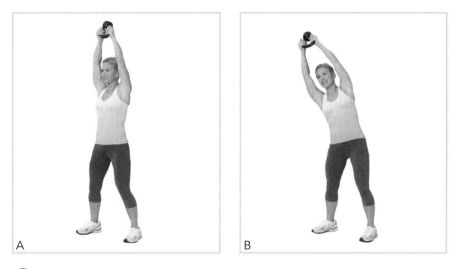

A   B

⌃ HALO

TARGETS ABS AND BACK

Hold the kettlebell upside down by the horns with both of your hands, arms overhead (A). Keeping your shoulders down, chest forward, and abs tight, rotate your torso from your waist in a circle to the left (B). The kettlebell should make small, controlled "halos" overhead. Repeat for 20 seconds (about six circles), then switch directions.

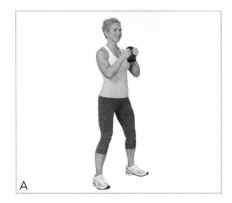
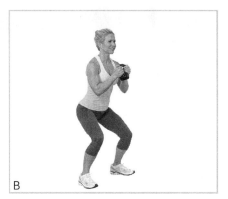

⌃ HALF SQUAT

TARGETS HIPS, BUTT, AND THIGHS

Hold the kettlebell by the horns with both of your hands in front of your chest (A). Shift your weight onto your heels, bend your knees and hips, and sit back, as if lowering halfway into a chair (B). Press into your heels and stand back up. Repeat for 40 seconds (about 40 squats).

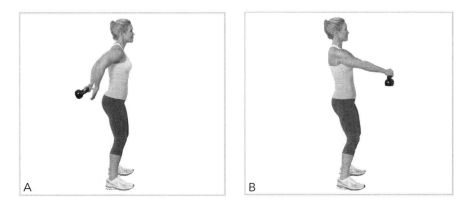

⌃ ROUND THE WORLD

TARGETS SHOULDERS AND ARMS

Hold the handle in your left hand, with your arms at your sides. Swing the weight around your back and pass the kettlebell to your right hand behind you (A). Continue circling around your front, passing the kettlebell back to your left hand (B). Repeat counterclockwise for 20 seconds (about 12 circles). Switch directions for another 20 seconds.

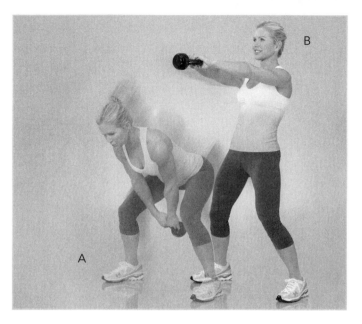

⌃ SQUAT AND SWING

TARGETS HIPS, BUTT, AND THIGHS

Stand with your feet more than hip-width apart and hold the handle with both of your hands, with your arms down and your palms in. Sit back into a squat (A). Then press into your heels, straighten your legs, and thrust your hips explosively upward to swing the kettlebell up to shoulder height (B). Keep your wrists in line with your forearms. (Your arms and shoulders should move as levers, rising and falling with momentum, as your hips do the work.) As the weight swings back between your legs, squat. Repeat for 1 minute (about 45 swings). Next do single-arm swings, passing the kettlebell from hand to hand at the top of each swing, for 1 minute (about 44 swings).

Make it easier: Use a lighter kettlebell (or dumbbell) or no weight at all.

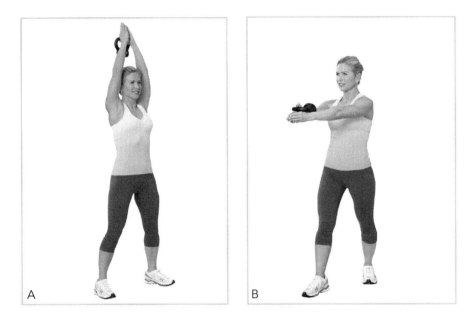

A

B

⌃ PIVOT AND POINT

TARGETS SHOULDERS AND BACK

Stand with your feet hip-width apart, palms together (prayer position) with the handle hooked over your thumbs, arms extended overhead (A). Pivot to the right on your heels so your right leg is lined up in front of your left leg. (Keep your head up, shoulders back, abs tight, and back straight.) At the same time, lower your arms to shoulder height (the base will rest on your wrists) (B). Turn back to the center, raising your arms overhead. Repeat for the left side. Alternate sides for 1 minute (about 20 reps).

Make it easier: Skip the overhead portion. Hold the weight in front of your chest and extend your arms to point to the side as you pivot.

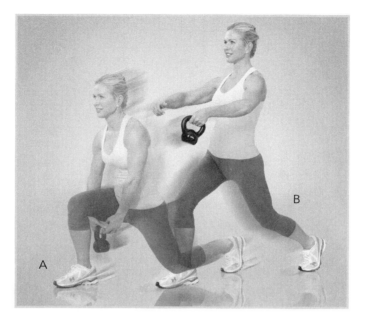

⌃ LUNGE AND LOOP

TARGETS ARMS, ABS, BUTT, AND LEGS

Hold the handle in your right hand, with your arms at your sides, palms in. Stand with your right foot 2 to 3 feet in front of your left, with your toes pointing forward, back heel off the floor. Bend your knees, lowering toward the floor, as you pass the kettlebell under your front leg to your left hand (A). Then pass it over your leg to your right hand as you straighten your legs (B). Continue for 30 seconds (about 18 loops), then reverse your arm direction for 30 seconds. Switch legs and repeat.

Make it easier: Just pass the weight back and forth underneath your leg each time you lunge instead of looping over the top.

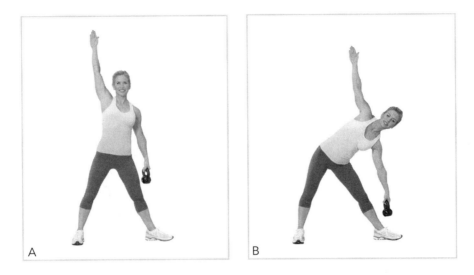

A

B

⊙ WINDMILL

TARGETS SHOULDERS, BACK, AND ABS

Hold the handle in your left hand and stand with your legs wide, with your left foot pointing to the side and your right one forward. Extend your right arm overhead, with your left arm at your side (A). Bend at the waist to the left and lower the kettlebell toward your left shin (B). Imagine that you are standing between two panes of glass to keep your body in line; don't roll forward or back. Slowly stand up, using your core muscles to lift. Repeat for 1 minute (about 20 reps), then switch sides.

Make it easier: Use a lighter kettlebell (or dumbbell) or no weight at all.

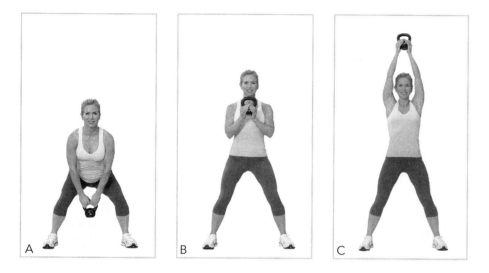

⌃ SQUAT, CATCH, AND PRESS

TARGETS SHOULDERS, ARMS, BUTT, AND LEGS

Stand with your feet more than hip-width apart and hold the handle with both of your hands, with your arms extended toward the floor. Sit back into a squat (A), then press into your heels and stand up. Use the momentum created by the hip thrust to help pull the weight up. (Your elbows will bend out to the sides as you lift the bell.) As the weight reaches your chest height, slide your hands down to grab the base (a slight tossing motion) (B). Press the weight overhead (C), then lower it to the starting position, sliding your hands back to the handle. Repeat for 1 minute (about 20 reps).

Make it easier: Don't press the kettlebell overhead.

CHAPTER 11

Your Body's Fat Traps—Beaten

Lose weight faster and keep it off with this breakthrough plan that derails your hunger and supercharges your workouts

Before you launch into yet another slim-down plan, beware: Your workouts may be working against you. In a study from the United Kingdom, some new exercisers compensated for their workouts by eating as much as 270 extra calories a day—negating more than half of the calories they burned. This self-sabotage has a ripple effect. As the number on the scale inches down at a painfully slow pace, many people give up altogether.

For women, there's an extra factor in the working-out-for-weight-loss equation: Women's bodies are designed to stubbornly hang on to fat, possibly to maintain their ability to reproduce. A study in the journal *Appetite* found that for every pound of fat women lost while dieting, their desire to eat increased about 2 percent. Exercise might trigger other defense mechanisms.

RESET YOUR HUNGER CLOCK

Time your meals to offset any exercise-induced desire to eat. One study found that appetite was suppressed longer when cyclists ate 1 hour before a 50-minute bike ride, compared with eating afterward.

Morning Exerciser

PREWORKOUT: Working out after an all-night fast can leave you feeling sluggish and ravenous. Instead, eat a little something, like 6 ounces low-fat yogurt with ½ cup chopped fruit (150 calories), 30 to 60 minutes before exercising. Can't stomach food that early? Opt for 8 ounces juice (122 calories).

POSTWORKOUT: Eat a small breakfast that includes carbs and protein within an hour of exercise to replenish energy stores. Try two eggs and toast (250 calories), 1 cup oatmeal with 2 tablespoons peanut butter (230 calories), or 1 cup cereal with low-fat or soy milk (177 calories).

Lunchtime Exerciser

PREWORKOUT: Going to a noon fitness class but haven't eaten since 8:00 a.m.? Try a cup of soup (about 150 calories) that has protein (chicken or beans) and carbohydrates (noodles or rice). It will also help hydrate you.

POSTWORKOUT: Eat the heavier part of your lunch. Good protein and fiber choices include peanut butter and banana on whole grain bread (337 calories) or chicken or turkey salad with extra veggies (285 calories).

After-Work Exerciser

PREWORKOUT: You'll be slacking if you go all afternoon without eating. Around 4:00 p.m., have a snack such as homemade trail mix (¼ cup nuts and ½ ounce raisins; 206 calories) or an apple with 2 teaspoons almond butter (160 calories).

POSTWORKOUT: Try to have dinner within an hour of working out. Studies show that exercisers who had to wait an hour or more before eating tended to consume more compared with those in studies in which meals were served sooner.

When sedentary overweight women exercised for over an hour 4 days in a row, levels of appetite hormones changed in ways that are likely to stimulate eating (the opposite was found in men), according to a University of Massachusetts study. And these studies don't take into account psychological saboteurs, such as rewarding yourself with dessert after a tough workout or toasting yourself with a glass of wine after a long day.

But here's the good news: You're not destined to succumb to your body's stay-fat traps. While half of new exercisers in the UK study ate more, the rest showed no signs of feeling hungrier, ate 130 fewer calories a day, and lost more than four times as much weight during the 12-week study. The first step is to know what you're up against; working out doesn't entitle you to eat whatever you want. Next, you need a smart exercise plan that curbs your hunger, coupled with an eating plan (see page 110) that fuels your workouts, not your appetite, so you don't take in calories you just burned off.

EASY-DOES-IT EXERCISE

When it comes to workouts that fight hunger, less may be better—at least in the beginning. In a Louisiana State University study, researchers discovered that overweight women who did an average of 60 minutes of easy exercise three times a week lost less weight than expected based on their calorie burn, probably because they ate more, says Tim Church, MD, PhD, director of the Laboratory of Preventive Medicine at the university's Pennington Biomedical Research Center. Those who exercised an average of 25 or 45 minutes three times a week dropped more weight, showing that they did not compensate for their workouts.

That's why our 6-week plan (see page 104) starts with short, moderate-intensity workouts. Then you'll build up to longer, more vigorous routines to help keep pounds off over the long haul. You'll also practice yoga (see page 105), which has been shown to diminish binge eating by 51 percent. Experts suspect that yoga might help by increasing body awareness, so you're more sensitive to feeling full, and you're also less likely to mindlessly stuff yourself.

CURB-YOUR-APPETITE WORKOUT PLAN

Week 1

4 days: 15–20 minutes of moderate-intensity cardio (walking, cycling, or using an elliptical machine). You should be breathing a little heavier but able to carry on a conversation.

3 or more days: Yoga (see page 105)

Week 2

4 days: 20–25 minutes of moderate-intensity cardio

3 or more days: Yoga

Week 3

4 days: 25–30 minutes of moderate-intensity cardio

3 or more days: Yoga

Week 4

4 days: 30–35 minutes of moderate-intensity cardio

3 or more days: Yoga

Week 5

2 days: 35–40 minutes of moderate-intensity cardio

2 days: 30 minutes of interval cardio, alternating 30–60 seconds of high-intensity activity (going faster or increasing resistance or incline so it's difficult to carry on a conversation) with 1- to 2-minute recovery bouts at a moderate intensity

3 or more days: Yoga

Week 6

2 days: 40–45 minutes of moderate-intensity cardio

3 days: 30 minutes of interval cardio

3 or more days: Yoga

Week 7 and Beyond

After 6 weeks, you can maintain the level of activity if you're satisfied with your results. To lose more weight or bust a plateau, continue to increase your moderate workouts up to 60 minutes total and the interval workouts up to 45 minutes total.

CURB-YOUR-APPETITE YOGA

This flowing yoga routine was developed by Laura Madden, a yoga instructor and fitness director of the Scottsdale Resort and Athletic Club in Arizona. Hold each pose for three to five breaths, unless otherwise directed.

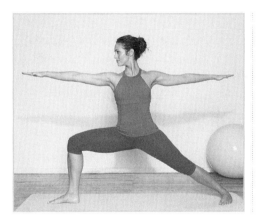

(<) WARRIOR II

Stand tall with your feet together. Take a large step to the right. Bend your right knee into a lunge, with your right knee over your ankle and your toes pointing to the right; point your left foot forward. Extend your arms out to the sides.

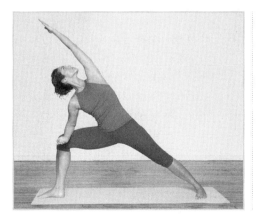

(<) SIDE REACH

From Warrior II, rest your right forearm on your thigh and reach your left arm overhead, lengthening your spine.

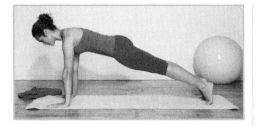

⊙ PLANK

From the Side Reach, place your hands on the floor, one on either side of your right foot. Move your right foot back next to your left one. Your hands should be directly beneath your shoulders; your body should be in a straight line from your head to your heels.

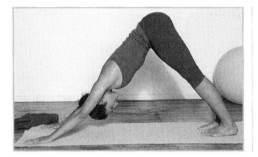

⊙ DOWNWARD-FACING DOG

From the Plank, reach your hips upward, bending your body into an upside-down V. Press your heels toward the floor.

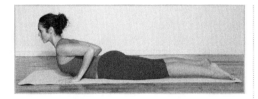

⊙ COBRA

From the Downward-Facing Dog, bend your knees and lower your body to the floor. With your hands under your shoulders, lift your chest off of the floor. Keep your shoulders down. Press your palms, hips, and tops of feet into the floor.

From Cobra, press up onto your knees, then your feet. Roll up one vertebra at a time so your head comes up last as you stand. Repeat the series, lunging to the left for moves 1 (Warrior II) and 2 (Side Reach). Once you've completed all five moves the second time, finish with the two on the opposite page.

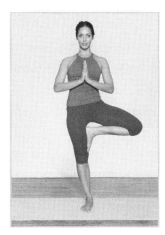

⟨<⟩ TREE POSE

Place your left foot against your right calf or inner thigh, not your knee. Lift your rib cage to elongate your spine, and bring your hands to a prayer position. Hold, then repeat with your opposite leg.

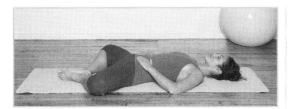

⟨<⟩ GODDESS POSE

Lie with the soles of your feet together and as close to your hips as comfortably possible, stretching your inner thighs. If this is too intense, straighten your legs. Breathe deeply in this pose for 2 to 5 minutes.

BREAK THE WORKOUT/PIG-OUT CYCLE

Working out can make you work up an appetite, but don't think you can indulge in fettuccine Alfredo or have ice cream every night as a reward. You'll lose more weight and see faster results if you combine exercise with the following smart eating strategies to curb your appetite. Here's how to avoid eating back all the calories you work off.

Eat every 3 or 4 hours. Giving your body a steady supply of calories keeps blood sugar normal during and after exercise, and it can prevent an excessively high insulin response the next time you eat that encourages excess body fat. To avoid taking in extra calories because you're eating more often, keep meals to 500 calories or less and snacks under 200, limiting total calories to about 1,600 to 1,800 a day.

Have protein at every meal. Protein increases satiety and helps keep your appetite under control by stimulating gut hormones that help you feel full. Options include eggs, milk, soy milk, yogurt, and oatmeal for breakfast. Include nuts, beans, whole grains, low-fat dairy, fish, lean meats, and poultry at other meals and snacks to ensure you get enough protein.

Load up on fiber. Bulky foods will fill you up on fewer calories. Aim for 25 to 30 grams of fiber per day. Include at least 5 grams in every meal and snack. At meals, try $\frac{1}{2}$ cup of black beans, 1 cup of split-pea soup, or 1 cup of steamed spinach with $\frac{1}{2}$ cup of raw carrot sticks. For snacks, try an apple plus a handful of nuts, or a rye crispbread and a pear.

Quench your thirst with water. Exercise is likely to increase your thirst, but many people mistake thirst for hunger. Next time you have the munchies, especially postworkout, try to satisfy your desire with calorie-free H_2O. Sipping sweetened drinks can quickly override any calorie deficit created by working out.

YOUR POST-PIG-OUT PLAN

So, you worked out, then pigged out. Don't stress out! Our 3-day program will help you turn back time. It's simple, fast, and effective. Stick with it and you will have those extra pounds gone.

BURN IT OFF, KEEP IT OFF

Here's how easy it is to negate your workout.

45 MINUTES OF . . .	BURNS . . .	ABOUT THE SAME AMOUNT IN . . .
Hatha yoga	128 calories*	5 oz red wine
Walking (3 mph)	168 calories	1 Luna Chocolate Raspberry bar
Brisk walking (4 mph)	255 calories	1 Snickers bar (2 oz)
Pilates	270 calories	1 Starbucks Venti Caffè Mocha with fat-free milk
Power yoga	310 calories	1 Häagen-Dazs Vanilla & Almonds ice cream bar
Slow jogging (5 mph)	408 calories	8 Oreo cookies
Spinning	459 calories	1 plain bagel with cream cheese
Elliptical trainer	488 calories	1 large McDonald's fries
Running (7 mph)	587 calories	1 large broccoli Cheddar soup at Au Bon Pain + 1 small caffè latte

*Based on a 150-pound person

Break the Cycle

The splurge: Too many sweet treats. While experts used to dismiss the notion of sugar addiction, a growing body of research suggests that the sweet stuff can hijack the same brain circuitry that's affected by drugs and alcohol, leading to a vicious cycle of cravings and binges. The sugar hooks you, while the fat piles on the pounds.

The solution: Eliminate desserts that are rich in sugar and fat for at least 3 days; 7 to 10 would be even better. This will help quell cravings while you reestablish a taste for naturally sweet foods such as fruit and starchy vegetables.

Resize Your Belly

The splurge: As the "I worked out; I deserve it" mentality sets in, one of your natural appetite control systems—the stomach's network of stretch receptors—starts losing its effectiveness. Normally, when your stomach is full, these receptors send messages to the brain that say "I'm satisfied." But prolonged periods of overeating make the receptors less sensitive. This helps explain why that feeling of "I'm so full; I'll never eat again" is followed the next day by the sense that you're even hungrier than usual.

The solution: If you keep eating the same high-calorie foods but merely reduce the quantity, your stretch receptors will signal your brain that you're starving and need emergency rations—now. But you can short-circuit this by eating healthy-size servings of low-calorie, high-fiber foods such as fruits, vegetables, and whole grains. Their bulk will keep the receptors happy while avoiding excess calories.

Cut Down on Cocktails

The splurge: The problem with alcohol isn't just the sugar. The alcohol itself packs in 7 calories per gram (compared with 4 for protein and carbs and 9 for fat). And the stomach and brain don't register liquid calories in the same way they do solids, so it's easy to go right on eating and drinking—without compensating for the added calories.

The solution: Satisfying, low-calorie beverages can boost metabolism and even temper your hunger. Tea (lose the cream and sugar) has zero calories and lifts metabolic rate. Or prepare a pitcher of flavored water. Add sliced oranges, lemons, and limes to a pitcher—or toss in berries or sprigs of mint or lemongrass. They're refreshing and give you healing antioxidants.

YOUR 3-DAY DETOX DIET

Now that you know the principles, you're ready to undo the damage. Our plan provides about 1,250 calories a day. To cut the craving for sweets, we've eliminated most refined sugars. To keep your stretch receptors happy, we feature plant-based foods that are rich in fiber. And instead of high-calorie cocktails, we give you delicious low- or no-cal drinks. If you're not back to your normal weight in 3 days, repeat for a total of 6 days.

Day 1

Breakfast

❑ Egg white–veggie scramble: ½ cup egg whites (or 4 egg whites) with 1 cup chopped mixed vegetables, prepared with cooking spray

❑ 1 slice toasted whole grain bread with 2 teaspoons 100 percent fruit spread

❑ 1 cup fat-free Greek-style yogurt

❑ Coffee or tea with ¼ cup fat-free milk

Morning Snack

❑ 1 sheet graham cracker with 2 teaspoons natural (no added sugar) peanut butter

Lunch

❑ Hummus-veggie pita sandwich: ½ whole grain pita spread with 1 teaspoon deli mustard and 1 tablespoon hummus, stuffed with vegetables and 2 slices avocado

❑ 1 medium orange or 2 tangerines

❑ Unsweetened herbal tea (hot or iced) with cinnamon stick

Afternoon Snack

❑ 1 cup mixed vegetables with 2 teaspoons oil and vinegar dressing

Dinner

❑ 3 ounces grilled salmon brushed with citrus glaze while cooking (1 tablespoon each orange juice, honey, and reduced-sodium soy sauce)

❑ ½ cup cooked brown rice prepared with 1 teaspoon olive oil

❑ 1 cup cooked winter squash, broccoli, or asparagus

Dessert

❑ ½ cup fat-free plain Greek-style yogurt with 2 teaspoons 100% fruit spread

Total: 1,288 calories, 91 g protein, 181 g carbohydrates, 26 g total fat, 4.5 g saturated fat, 27 g dietary fiber, 1,322 mg sodium, 82 mg cholesterol

Day 2

Breakfast

❏ 1 cup low-fat (1 percent), no-added-salt cottage cheese with ½ cup pineapple chunks

❏ 5 whole grain crackers

❏ Coffee or tea with ¼ cup fat-free milk

Morning Snack

❏ ½ turkey sandwich: 1 slice whole grain bread with 2 ounces low-sodium or reduced-sodium turkey breast, lettuce, tomato, and 1 teaspoon mustard

Lunch

❏ Pasta tuna salad: 1 cup cooked whole grain pasta spirals or bow ties with 1 cup chopped cherry tomatoes and tuna salad (4 ounces water-packed tuna mixed with 2 tablespoons chopped white onion, 1 tablespoon fat-free Greek-style yogurt, and 2 teaspoons Dijon mustard)

❏ Water with sprigs of mint or lemongrass

Afternoon Snack

❏ 1 medium orange

Dinner

❏ 3 ounces broiled or grilled boneless chicken breast

❏ 1 medium baked sweet potato topped with 2 teaspoons light spread

❏ 2 cups tossed field greens drizzled with 1 tablespoon vinaigrette dressing

❏ Unsweetened herbal tea (hot or iced) with lemon

Total: 1,242 calories, 122 g protein, 146 g carbohydrates, 21.5 g total fat, 4 g saturated fat, 26 g dietary fiber, 1,565 mg sodium

Day 3

Breakfast

❑ 1 cup cooked oatmeal topped with ¼ cup fat-free plain or vanilla Greek-style yogurt and 1 cup berries

❑ Coffee or tea with ¼ cup fat-free milk

Morning Snack

❑ 1 ounce low-fat cheese with 5 whole grain crackers

Lunch

❑ 1 cup low-sodium lentil soup or minestrone soup

❑ 2 cups mixed salad greens with ¼ cup low-sodium water-packed tuna or low-sodium diced turkey and 1 teaspoon olive oil with lemon juice or balsamic vinegar

❑ Unsweetened herbal tea with cinnamon stick

Afternoon Snack

❑ 1 piece fresh fruit (banana or apple) or 1 cup berries, with 8 ounces fat-free plain or vanilla Greek-style yogurt

Dinner

❑ Veggie burger on whole wheat bun topped with 2 slices avocado

❑ Spinach salad: 1½ cups baby spinach; ¼ red onion, sliced; ¼ cup fresh mandarin orange slices; and 1 teaspoon olive oil with balsamic vinegar

❑ Seltzer water with sliced lemon, orange, or lime

Total: 1,277 calories, 86 g protein, 173 g carbohydrates, 32 g total fat, 5 g saturated fat, 34 g dietary fiber, 1,577 mg sodium

journal

"I'M NINE SIZES SMALLER!"

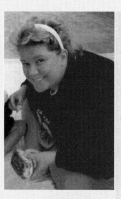

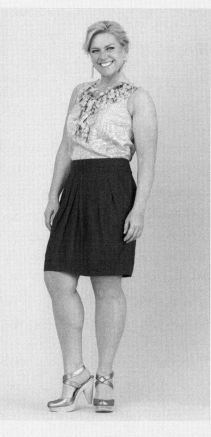

By cutting out soda and leaning on my personal-trainer sis for help, I got fit for life

by Sheri Harkness

My parents divorced during my junior year of high school, and I ate to soothe my emotions. In my twenties, two pregnancies packed on more weight. I made sure that my boys ate balanced meals, but I opted for greasy takeout and liters of soda. By age 35, I weighed almost 300 pounds.

Good-Bye, Gimmicks!

I was no stranger to weight-loss fads. My younger sister Karen, a personal trainer, encouraged me to get fit once and for all, but it wasn't until I stepped on the scale for a physical and weighed in at 282 pounds that I realized I had to change. I devised a strategy: I'd eat the same foods but halve the portions. I also gave up the 2 liters of soda I was guzzling each day.

About 2 weeks after I cut my food intake, I decided to go to the gym just 3 afternoons a week and walk on the treadmill for 15 minutes. Soon I was walking 4 days a week—and, finally, using the elliptical for an hour to burn 700 calories! After 2 months of building up my stamina with cardio, I turned to Karen for help. She e-mailed me loads of weight-training workouts, including photos of the specific machines. Soon my body became toned for the first time in my life.

In February 2009, I participated in the Empire State Building Run-Up, a race where thousands climb the 86 floors up to the observatory deck. I couldn't believe how far I had come, bounding up scores of steps when just months before I could barely walk on the treadmill. Losing 141 pounds in just 18 months was (and still is!) an incredible feeling.

Here are my top tips:

FIND A MANTRA. Mine is "Never give up." It helped keep me on track!

WATCH FOR SNEAKY DIET SABOTEURS. I did the math and realized that I drank 260,000 calories—or 74 pounds' worth of empty calories—per year in soda alone. That was a huge eye-opener!

MAKE IT ABOUT YOUR HEALTH. My sister taught me to focus on my overall fitness rather than just a number on the scale. She was right: When I learned to love exercise and set goals at the gym, the weight loss that followed was just an added bonus.

LEARN TO APPRECIATE REAL FOOD. I stopped viewing food as recreation and began to see it as fuel. These days, I've given up takeout and try to buy natural whenever possible. No matter what, I'll always fall back on grilled chicken, salads, whole grain cereals, and fruit.

Bonus Weight-Loss
COOKBOOK

On the pages that follow, you'll find *Prevention's* best recipes to help you lose weight and look great. They're delicious, nutritious, and quick and easy, too.

35 DELICIOUS RECIPES

BREAKFASTS

SALADS AND SOUPS

SIDE DISHES

MAIN DISHES

DESSERTS

GINGERED CANTALOUPE SMOOTHIE

MAKES 4 SERVINGS

20 ice cubes

2 cups cubed cantaloupe
(about ½ melon)

6 ounces low-fat plain yogurt

3 tablespoons sugar

½ teaspoon grated fresh
ginger

In a blender, combine the ice cubes, cantaloupe,
yogurt, sugar, and ginger and puree until
smooth. Taste and add more sugar if you like.

PER SERVING: 91 calories, 3 g protein, 19 g
carbohydrates, 1 g total fat, 0.5 g saturated fat, 1 g dietary
fiber, 46 mg sodium

BLUEBERRY-POMEGRANATE SMOOTHIE

MAKES 1 SERVING

⅔ cup frozen blueberries
(not thawed)

½ cup fat-free French vanilla
yogurt (We used Stonyfield.)

⅓ cup vanilla soy milk (We
used Silk.)

¼ cup pomegranate juice
(100% pure juice)

In a blender, place the blueberries, yogurt, milk,
and juice. Blend on high speed until smooth.

PER SERVING: 227 calories, 9 g protein, 45 g
carbohydrates, 2 g total fat, 0.5 g saturated fat, 3 g dietary
fiber, 123 mg sodium

100

THE PERCENTAGE OF THE DAILY
REQUIREMENT FOR VITAMINS A AND C
IN HALF A CANTALOUPE

MINTED YOGURT PARFAIT

MAKES 4 SERVINGS

2½ cups fresh blueberries

2 tablespoons chopped fresh mint

2 tablespoons honey

1 teaspoon freshly grated orange peel (from 1 orange), optional

¼ cup pecans, toasted and coarsely chopped

1 cup vanilla frozen yogurt

In a bowl, toss together the blueberries, mint, honey, orange peel (if using), and 3 tablespoons of the pecans. Spoon about half of the berry mixture into 4 glasses. Top each with 2 tablespoons of the frozen yogurt. Divide the remaining berries among the glasses and top each with 2 more tablespoons yogurt. Sprinkle with the remaining pecans.

PER SERVING: 213 calories, 6 g protein, 34 g carbohydrates, 7 g total fat, 2 g saturated fat, 3 g dietary fiber, 29 mg sodium

GINGERSNAP OATMEAL

MAKES 1 SERVING

½ cup apple juice

¼ cup water

¼ quick-cooking steel-cut oats (We used McCann's Quick & Easy.)

1 roughly broken gingersnap

1 tablespoon chopped pecans

Chopped fresh fruit (optional)

In a small, heavy saucepan, bring the juice and water to a boil. Add the oats, reduce the heat to low, and simmer uncovered for 5 minutes, stirring often.

Remove from the heat and let stand for 2 minutes. Spoon into a serving bowl and sprinkle with the gingersnap and pecans. Garnish with the fruit (if using).

PER SERVING: 283 calories, 5 g protein, 46 g carbohydrates, 8 g total fat, 1 g saturated fat, 5 g dietary fiber, 53 mg sodium

FRUIT-GRANOLA CRUMBLE

MAKES 6 SERVINGS

3 cups fresh blueberries

4 thinly sliced fresh peaches (about 1¼ pounds or 4 cups) or 1 pound frozen sliced peaches, thawed

⅓ cup sugar

2 tablespoons all-purpose flour

1 teaspoon ground ginger

½ teaspoon salt

1½ cups granola (without dried fruit), large pieces broken apart

½ cup walnut halves, chopped

1½ tablespoons butter

Preheat the oven to 375°F.

In an 8" × 8" pan, mix the blueberries and peaches.

In a bowl, combine the sugar, flour, ginger, and salt and then stir into the fruit. Top with the granola and walnuts and dot with the butter. Bake for about 45 minutes, until the fruit is bubbly. Cool for at least 5 minutes. Serve warm, at room temperature, or cold.

PER SERVING: 294 calories, 5 g protein, 49 g carbohydrates, 11 g total fat, 3 g saturated fat, 5 g dietary fiber, 256 mg sodium

SUNDAY MORNING BRUNCH WAFFLES

MAKES 8 SERVINGS

2 cups strawberries, sliced

1 cup raspberries

1 cup blueberries or blackberries

1 package (4-serving size) fat-free, sugar-free instant vanilla pudding

2¼ cups cold 1% milk

1 tablespoon grated lemon zest

2 tablespoons lemon juice

1 cup thawed light frozen whipped topping

8 small Belgian or regular frozen waffles, toasted

In a small bowl, combine the strawberries, raspberries, and blueberries or blackberries. Set aside.

Whisk together the pudding, milk, lemon zest, and lemon juice for 2 minutes, or until well blended. Gently stir in the whipped topping.

Place ¼ cup of the pudding mixture on each of 8 plates. Top each with a waffle. Spoon the fruit over each and drizzle with the remaining pudding.

PER SERVING: 295 calories, 7 g protein, 49 g carbohydrates, 9 g total fat, 3 g saturated fat, 4 g dietary fiber, 579 mg sodium

SUPERFOOD: BLUEBERRIES

B lueberries are abundant (and cheap!) in the United States, especially in the summer months of June through August. Packed with antioxidants, vitamin C, manganese, and fiber, blueberries might promote brain health by improving learning and keeping memory sharp.

Look for berries that still have their silver-white surface bloom. The light coating indicates freshness and helps keep juices in. The fruit should move around easily when you jiggle a pint, a sign that no soft or moldy berries are stuck together.

FALL FRITTATA

MAKES 6 SERVINGS

1 small onion, chopped

4 tablespoons olive oil

12 small potatoes (10 ounces)

½ teaspoon salt

2 cloves garlic, minced

5 cups spinach (about 4 ounces)

8 large eggs, beaten

Freshly ground black pepper

3 tablespoons grated Parmesan cheese

In a nonstick, ovenproof skillet, cook the onion in 2 tablespoons of the oil.

Thinly slice the potatoes and add with ¼ teaspoon of the salt. Cook for 10 minutes, stirring occasionally. Add the garlic and cook until the potatoes are done. Stir in the spinach until wilted. Transfer to a bowl to cool. Stir in the eggs, ¼ teaspoon of the salt, and pepper to taste.

In the same pan, heat the remaining 2 tablespoons oil over medium-low heat. Cook the egg mixture, sprinkled with the cheese, until almost set. Broil briefly to brown.

PER SERVING: 233 calories, 11 g protein, 11 g carbohydrates, 16 g total fat, 4 g saturated fat, 2 g dietary fiber, 344 mg sodium

CREAMY ITALIAN PASTA SALAD

MAKES 4 SERVINGS

2 cups whole grain rotini

½ cup 0% plain Greek yogurt

2 tablespoons Parmesan cheese

2 tablespoons chopped fresh basil

1 tablespoon red wine vinegar

½ teaspoon dried mustard

1 clove garlic, minced

1 can (6 ounces) solid white tuna packed in water, drained and flaked

4 cups chopped romaine

1 cup cherry tomatoes, halved

Prepare the pasta according to package directions. Rinse under cold water and drain.

Meanwhile, in a large bowl, stir together the yogurt, cheese, basil, vinegar, mustard, and garlic. Add the tuna, romaine, tomatoes, and pasta. Toss to coat well.

PER SERVING: 283 calories, 6 g protein, 45 g carbohydrates, 3 g total fat, 1 g saturated fat, 6 g dietary fiber, 232 mg sodium

FRUITY SALAD

MAKES 4 SERVINGS

1½ tablespoons olive oil

1 tablespoon red wine vinegar

¼ teaspoon salt

⅛ teaspoon freshly ground black pepper

4 cups baby spinach (about 4 ounces)

1 pear (such as Bosc), peeled, cored, halved lengthwise, and thinly sliced

½ cup dried cranberries

¼ cup walnut pieces, toasted

¼ cup thinly sliced red onion

In a large bowl, whisk together the oil, vinegar, salt, and pepper. Add the spinach, pear, cranberries, walnuts, and onion and toss. Season to taste with additional salt and pepper.

PER SERVING: 182 calories, 2 g protein, 24 g carbohydrates, 10 g total fat, 1 g saturated fat, 4 g dietary fiber, 192 mg sodium

SUPERFOOD: SPINACH

TASTE IT: Greens thrive in cool weather, so local spinach is the most flavorful and affordable in September and October and March through May.

LOVE IT: Popeye was right. Spinach is a powerhouse, loaded with vitamins, antioxidants, and essential nutrients. It's one of the healthiest foods in the world, topping most other vegetables.

STORE IT: Keep spinach in the crisper drawer, loosely wrapped in paper towels and tucked in a plastic bag (just folded shut, not sealed).

AUTUMN SALAD

4 teaspoons olive oil

1 tablespoon white wine vinegar

2 teaspoons honey

¼ teaspoon salt

⅛ teaspoon freshly ground black pepper

3 medium sweet-tart apples (such as Braeburn), quartered and thinly sliced crosswise

1½ cups thinly sliced red cabbage

⅓ cup crumbled mild blue cheese

¼ cup thinly sliced red onion

¼ cup coarsely chopped toasted walnuts

In a large bowl, whisk together the oil, vinegar, honey, salt, and pepper. Add the apples, cabbage, cheese, onion, and walnuts. Toss to combine.

PER SERVING: 220 calories, 4 g protein, 26 g carbohydrates, 13 g total fat, 3 g saturated fat, 4 g dietary fiber, 311 mg sodium

18
THE PERCENTAGE OF THE DAILY REQUIREMENT FOR FIBER IN 1 MEDIUM APPLE

WARM SHRIMP
AND PINEAPPLE SALAD

MAKES 4 SERVINGS

1 package (16 ounces) frozen black-eyed peas (about 3¾ cups)

1¼ cups frozen green peas

½ red bell pepper, chopped

1 tablespoon olive oil

1 teaspoon paprika

½ teaspoon salt

1 pound large shrimp, peeled and cooked

1⅓ cups chopped pineapple

2 teaspoons lime juice

⅛ teaspoon hot-pepper sauce

⅓ cup fresh basil leaves, chopped (optional)

In a large pan, combine the black-eyed peas, green peas, bell pepper, oil, paprika, and salt and cook over medium-high heat for 4 minutes. Add the shrimp and cook for 2 minutes, until heated through. Toss in the pineapple, juice, hot-pepper sauce, and basil (if using). Season to taste with salt and pepper.

PER SERVING: 415 calories, 43 g protein, 47 g carbohydrates, 7 g total fat, 1 g saturated fat, 10 g dietary fiber, 579 mg sodium

HOT OR COLD PASTA SALAD

MAKES 4 SERVINGS

This pasta and veggie combination is all about convenience. You can serve this side dish however you like—warm, cold, or at room temperature. It's delicious no matter what!

2 tablespoons sliced almonds

6 ounces orzo (about 1 cup)

2 tablespoons olive oil

3 cloves garlic, finely chopped

⅛ teaspoon ground red pepper (optional)

1 pound asparagus, trimmed, cooked by any method, and cut diagonally into quarters

¾ teaspoon salt

1 tablespoon + 1 teaspoon lemon peel (from 2 lemons)

1 tablespoon lemon juice

¼ cup freshly grated Parmesan cheese

2 tablespoons dried cranberries

Freshly ground black pepper

Preheat the oven to 350°F.

Place the almonds on a baking pan and toast in the oven for 5 to 10 minutes, until browned.

Prepare the orzo according to the package directions and drain.

In a medium saucepan, heat the oil over medium-low heat. Add the garlic and red pepper (if using), and cook for about 3 minutes, until softened. Add the asparagus and heat through for about 2 minutes. Stir in the orzo and salt and toss to combine.

Remove from the heat. Add the lemon peel, lemon juice, Parmesan, and cranberries. Season to taste with salt and pepper. Top with the almonds just before serving.

PER SERVING: 281 calories, 10 g protein, 39 g carbohydrates, 10.5 g total fat, 2 g saturated fat, 3 g dietary fiber, 517 mg sodium

SPINACH AND TORTELLINI SOUP

MAKES 4 SERVINGS

A few flavorful ingredients are all it takes to whip up a warm, satisfying weeknight meal in a bowl.

4 cups chicken broth (We used Kitchen Basics.)

1 cup water

1 package (9 ounces) fresh cheese tortellini (We used Buitoni.)

6 ounces spinach

Salt

Freshly ground black pepper

Parmesan cheese

In a large saucepan, bring the broth and water to a boil. Reduce the heat, add the tortellini, and simmer until the pasta is tender, about 6 minutes. Stir in the spinach and cook until just wilted. Season with salt and pepper to taste. Ladle the soup into 4 bowls, and shave or grate the Parmesan over the top.

PER SERVING: 249 calories, 16 g protein, 36 g carbohydrates, 5 g total fat, 3 g saturated fat, 4 g dietary fiber, 839 mg sodium

ROASTED PEPPER AND SWEET CORN SOUP

MAKES 4 SERVINGS

4 cups roasted red pepper and tomato soup (We used Pacific Natural Foods Organic.)

1½ cups frozen sweet corn kernels

2 tablespoons basil pesto (Look for it in the refrigerated pasta case or pasta aisle.)

¼ cup low-fat plain Greek-style yogurt

In a large saucepan, combine the soup, corn, and pesto. Cover and bring just to boiling. Reduce the heat and simmer, partially covered, for 3 minutes. Ladle into 4 bowls and top each with a dollop of yogurt.

PER SERVING: 203 calories, 9 g protein, 27 g carbohydrates, 6 g total fat, 3 g saturated fat, 2 g dietary fiber, 784 mg sodium

STEAK, POTATO, AND VEGETABLE SOUP

MAKES 4 SERVINGS

1 tablespoon olive oil

1 pound beef stir-fry strips (Look for it in the meat case.)

2 tablespoons flour

¼ teaspoon salt

2 cups water

4 cups chicken broth (We used Kitchen Basics.)

2 cups refrigerated diced potatoes with onion (We used Simply Potatoes.)

2 cups frozen soup vegetables

1 tablespoon Worcestershire sauce

¼ teaspoon freshly ground black pepper

In a pot, heat the oil over medium-high heat. Add the beef and sprinkle with the flour. Cook, stirring, for 3 minutes or until browned. Add the salt. Stir in the water, scraping the bottom of the pot. Add the broth, potatoes, and vegetables. Reduce the heat. Simmer for 15 minutes, until the potatoes are tender. Add the Worcestershire sauce, pepper, and salt to taste.

PER SERVING: 323 calories, 33 g protein, 26 g carbohydrates, 9 g total fat, 2.5 g saturated fat, 3 g dietary fiber, 859 mg sodium

---

SUPERFOOD: PARSNIP!

Don't let its pale color fool you: A serving of this low-calorie veggie is packed with 7 grams of fiber (40 percent more than its brighter-colored cousin, the carrot), 30 micrograms of bone-building vitamin K, and 30 percent of the immune-boosting vitamin C you need daily.

Buy parsnips that are smooth, off-white, and firm and small to medium in size. Parsnip ripens after the first frost, so winter months are prime for buying. Store in the fridge.

Try parsnip peeled and diced. It's delicious cooked in soups and stews or raw in salads. For a healthy side, boil and mash them as you would potatoes. Their sweet, mild flavor requires less butter.

ITALIAN LENTIL AND BROCCOLI STEW

MAKES 4 SERVINGS

Red-pepper flakes add heat to this recipe, and oregano, onion, and garlic boost the taste even more. They transform earthy lentils and vitamin-rich broccoli into a succulent stew.

1 small onion, finely chopped

1 small carrot, finely chopped

2 cloves garlic, minced

2 teaspoons olive oil

2 cups reduced-sodium vegetable broth or water

1 cup dried green or brown lentils

1 teaspoon dried oregano

¼ teaspoon red-pepper flakes

6 cups broccoli florets

16 large pitted green olives, slivered

4 teaspoons shredded Parmesan cheese

In a medium saucepan, combine the onion, carrot, garlic, and oil. Cover and cook over medium heat for 5 minutes, or until the vegetables start to soften. Stir in the broth, lentils, oregano, and pepper flakes. Cover and bring almost to a boil. Reduce to a simmer and cook for about 20 minutes, until the lentils are tender.

Add the broccoli. Cover and simmer for about 5 minutes, until the broccoli is crisp-tender. Stir in the olives. Add more water, if necessary, to thin the stew to the desired consistency. Serve sprinkled with the cheese.

PER SERVING: 271 calories, 17 g protein, 38 g carbohydrates, 7 g total fat, 1 g saturated fat, 15 g dietary fiber, 313 mg sodium

SIDE DISHES

PICKLED RED BEET EGGS

MAKES 8 SERVINGS

This is a real Pennsylvania Dutch delicacy and beautiful to boot. They're a tasty addition to any salad.

6 red beets, trimmed (about 2 pounds trimmed)

8 cups water

1 cup apple cider vinegar

½ cup sugar

6 whole cloves

1 stick cinnamon

½ teaspoon salt

8 hard-cooked eggs, peeled

1 shallot, chopped (optional)

In a large pot, place the beets and water. Bring to a boil and cook for 30 minutes, or until tender. Remove the beets and let cool for 10 minutes.

Transfer 4 cups of the cooked red-beet juice to a saucepan and add the vinegar, sugar, cloves, cinnamon, and salt. Cook over medium heat for about 5 minutes, until the sugar is dissolved.

In a large bowl, combine the eggs, red-beet liquid mixture, and shallot (if using). Slip the skins off the cooled beets. Slice the beets and add to the bowl. Chill overnight.

PER SERVING: 159 calories, 7 g protein, 19 g carbohydrates, 6 g total fat, 1.5 g saturated fat, 2 g dietary fiber, 264 mg sodium

CHEESY SCALLOPED POTATOES

MAKES 8 SERVINGS

2 pounds all-purpose potatoes, peeled and thinly sliced

1¼ cups grated Cheddar cheese (5 ounces)

Salt

Freshly ground black pepper

¾ cup fat-free milk

2 tablespoons olive oil

Preheat the oven to 350°F. Set the oven rack to the top position.

In a well-oiled 8" × 8" baking dish, layer the potatoes and cheese, ending with the cheese on top. Season each potato layer with salt and pepper to taste. Pour in the milk, then drizzle the oil over the potatoes and cheese.

Bake on the top rack of the oven for 1 hour 15 minutes, or until bubbly and golden.

PER SERVING: 200 calories, 7 g protein, 23 g carbohydrates, 10 g total fat, 4 g saturated fat, 2 g dietary fiber, 125 mg sodium

MASHED SWEET POTATOES WITH APPLE JUICE

MAKES 4 SERVINGS

These potatoes keep in the refrigerator for up to 5 days.

2 pounds sweet potatoes (about 4), peeled and cut into large dice

⅔ cup apple juice

1 tablespoon butter

½ teaspoon salt

¼ teaspoon ground nutmeg

Large pinch of freshly ground black pepper

In a medium saucepan, bring the potatoes and juice to a boil. Reduce the heat and simmer, covered, stirring occasionally, for 25 minutes, or until the potatoes are soft enough to mash.

In a food processor, put the potatoes and juice. Add the butter, salt, nutmeg, and pepper, and puree. Taste and add more salt and pepper if you like.

PER SERVING: 180 calories, 2 g protein, 36 g carbohydrates, 10 g total fat, 2 g saturated fat, 4 g dietary fiber, 360 mg sodium

SUPERFOOD: APPLES

An apple juice a day might keep the doctor away, according to a Spanish study. When researchers used a new, more accurate technique to analyze the levels of vitamin C in 17 fruit juices and soft drinks, apple juice came out on top—beating orange juice by as much as 14 milligrams per ounce. Extra ascorbic acid might have been added to the apple juices during production to increase levels of vitamin C, say researchers. Look for 100 percent apple juice (with no additional sweeteners), and stick to 8 ounces.

ASPARAGUS AND SUGAR SNAP TOSS

1½ teaspoons olive oil

1½ pounds asparagus, trimmed and cut into 1" pieces

1 tablespoon water

½ pound sugar snap peas, ends trimmed and strings removed

3 scallions, sliced

1½ teaspoons reduced-sodium soy sauce

1½ teaspoons honey

Salt

Freshly ground black pepper

In a large pan with a lid, heat the oil over medium heat. Add the asparagus and water. Cover and steam for 5 minutes.

Add the peas, scallions, soy sauce, and honey. Cover and cook until tender, for about 5 minutes.

Season to taste with salt and pepper and serve warm or at room temperature.

PER SERVING: 34 calories, 2 g protein, 5 g carbohydrates, 1 g total fat, 0 g saturated fat, 2 g dietary fiber, 36 mg sodium

GRILLED SPINACH

MAKES 4 SERVINGS

Steaming this spinach in a foil pouch concentrates the flavors and preserves the nutrients.

12 ounces fresh spinach, large stems removed

¼ teaspoon salt

Freshly ground black pepper

½ teaspoon sesame seeds (optional)

Preheat the grill or broiler. Cut an 18" × 18" square of heavy-duty foil or arrange 2 narrower lengths in a cross shape. Spray with oil.

Place the spinach on the foil, spray with oil, and toss with the salt. Fold over the foil and seal the edges to form a well-sealed pouch. Cook until the spinach is wilted, about 10 minutes. Season to taste with salt and freshly ground black pepper. Top with sesame seeds (if using).

PER SERVING: 20 calories, 2 g protein, 3 g carbohydrates, 1 g total fat, 0 g saturated fat, 2 g dietary fiber, 213 mg sodium

ROASTED ARTICHOKE TOSS

MAKES 4 SERVINGS

8 baby artichokes

½ lemon

1½ tablespoons olive oil

1 medium red onion, sliced

2 cloves garlic, halved

½ teaspoon salt

½ cup water

2 tablespoons balsamic vinegar

Preheat the oven to 400°F.

Halve the artichokes lengthwise, trim ½" from the leaves, scrape out the chokes, and rub the outsides with the lemon.

In a large ovenproof skillet, heat the oil over medium heat. Add the artichokes, onion, garlic, and salt. Brown lightly for 8 minutes. Add the water. Cover and bake for 20 minutes. Uncover and roast for 10 minutes, until the flesh of the leaves is tender. Splash with the vinegar.

PER SERVING: 129 calories, 4 g protein, 19 g carbohydrates, 6 g total fat, 1 g saturated fat, 11 g dietary fiber, 367 mg sodium

SUPERFOOD: ARTICHOKES

These versatile green globes (sometimes with a violet tinge) are fun to eat and full of flavor, whether they're full-size or "baby" versions. You'll find artichokes, which supply heart-healthy fiber, folate, and antioxidants, in markets year-round, but their peak season is May. Choose ones with tightly closed leaves; avoid artichokes that look dry or brown. Store them in an airtight plastic bag in the refrigerator for up to 5 days.

MAIN DISHES

SPEEDY CHEESESTEAK

MAKES 4 SERVINGS

Satisfy a hearty appetite with lean meat and real cheese, rather than processed. Buy your deli's best roast beef and provolone, plus bakery rolls and precut onions and peppers for a taste that beats takeout.

4 steak rolls (Look for them in the bakery or bread aisle.)

4 teaspoons olive oil

1 cup precut onions and bell peppers

Salt

Freshly ground black pepper

¾ pound sliced roast beef

4 slices provolone cheese

Preheat the broiler.

Brush the cut sides of the rolls with the oil. Toast in the broiler.

Meanwhile, in a small nonstick skillet, heat the oil over medium heat. Add the onions and bell peppers, season with salt and pepper, and cook until tender and browned.

Divide the roast beef among the bottom halves of the rolls. Top with the vegetables. Put a slice of cheese on the top halves of the rolls. Broil the sandwich halves for about 2 minutes, until heated through and the cheese browns slightly.

PER SERVING: 406 calories, 31 g protein, 33 g carbohydrates, 15 g total fat, 6 g saturated fat, 2 g dietary fiber, 535 mg sodium

CHICKEN CACCIATORE

MAKES 4 SERVINGS

Basil and oregano give the lead herbal notes here. Our version of Chicken Cacciatore cooks faster because the chicken is cut into small pieces, and the added pasta makes it a complete meal.

4 ounces multigrain rotini pasta

2 teaspoons olive oil

1 pound boneless, skinless chicken breast tenders, cut into ½" pieces

1 package (8 ounces) brown mushrooms (cremini), quartered

½ medium red bell pepper, cut into strips

1 small onion, chopped

2 cloves garlic, minced

¼ teaspoon salt

¼ teaspoon freshly ground black pepper

1 can (14.5 ounces) no-salt-added basil-garlic-oregano diced tomatoes

20 large pitted black olives

1 tablespoon finely chopped fresh parsley

Prepare the pasta according to the package directions.

Meanwhile, in a large nonstick skillet (with cover), heat the oil over medium-high heat. Add the chicken and cook, turning occasionally, for about 4 minutes, until browned on all sides. Transfer to a bowl.

In the pan, combine the mushrooms, bell pepper, onion, garlic, salt, and black pepper. Reduce the heat to medium, cover, and cook, stirring occasionally, for 3 minutes, or until the mushrooms exude liquid. Uncover and cook for about 8 minutes, until most of the liquid evaporates.

Stir in the tomatoes (with juice) and reserved chicken with any accumulated juices from the bowl. Reduce the heat to a simmer.

Add the drained pasta to the pan. Add the olives and toss gently to combine. Serve sprinkled with the parsley.

PER SERVING: 322 calories, 33 g protein, 34 g carbohydrates, 7 g total fat, 1 g saturated fat, 6 g dietary fiber, 460 mg sodium

PULLED PORK PIZZA

MAKES 4 SERVINGS

Barbecue sauce and heat-and-serve pulled pork give this superfast pizza a tangy taste that's deliciously different. A prebaked crust and shredded cheese save time and effort. Toss a simple salad while the pizza cooks to round out the meal.

1 prebaked thin pizza crust (We used Boboli Thin Crust.)

¼ cup + 2 tablespoons barbecue sauce

½ cup heat-and-serve pulled pork (We used Jack Daniel's.)

1 cup shredded mozzarella and provolone cheese blend (We used Sargento.)

Preheat the oven to 450°F.

Put the pizza crust on a pizza pan or large baking sheet. Lightly brush the crust with ¼ cup of the barbecue sauce. Scatter the pulled pork on top. Brush the remaining 2 tablespoons barbecue sauce over the meat. Sprinkle with the cheese. Bake for 8 to 10 minutes, until heated through and the cheese melts.

PER SERVING: 386 calories, 17 g protein, 47 g carbohydrates, 14 g total fat, 6 g saturated fat, 2 g dietary fiber, 1,072 mg sodium

LINGUINE BOLOGNESE

MAKES 4 SERVINGS

With tomatoes and tomato paste forming the base of the sauce and oregano, onion, and garlic layered on top, you'll never guess how little sauce is in this yummy pasta with meat sauce.

6 ounces whole wheat linguine

8 ounces extra-lean ground beef

1 medium onion, chopped

¼ cup chopped carrot

2 cloves garlic, minced

1 teaspoon dried oregano

1 medium zucchini, chopped

1 can (14.5 ounces) no-salt-added diced tomatoes

½ cup unsalted tomato paste

¼ cup water

¼ teaspoon salt

3 tablespoons shredded part-skim mozzarella

Prepare the pasta according to the package directions.

Heat a large nonstick skillet over medium-high heat. Add the beef and cook, breaking the meat into smaller pieces, for 3 or 4 minutes, until no longer pink. Stir in the onion, carrot, garlic, and oregano. Cook, stirring occasionally, for about 2 minutes, until the vegetables start to soften. Add the zucchini and cook another 2 minutes, until it starts to soften. Stir in the tomatoes (with juice), tomato paste, and water. Bring to a boil, reduce the heat to medium, and simmer for 12 to 15 minutes, until slightly thickened. Remove from the heat and stir in the salt.

Serve the sauce over the drained pasta, and sprinkle with the cheese.

PER SERVING: 302 calories, 22 g protein, 48 g carbohydrates, 4 g total fat, 2 g saturated fat, 9 g dietary fiber, 268 mg sodium

SALMON WITH A TWIST

A delicious, nutritious dinner doesn't get much easier than this—and only one pan to clean! Salmon topped with a creamy Parmesan sauce roasts in the oven alongside a medley of green beans and corn.

12 ounces trimmed fresh green beans

½ teaspoon olive oil

Salt

Freshly ground black pepper

2 cups frozen corn kernels

4 4- to 6-ounce skinless salmon fillets

¼ cup mayonnaise

¼ cup shredded Parmesan cheese

Preheat the oven to 450°F. Coat a rimmed baking sheet with cooking spray.

Place the beans on the baking sheet. Drizzle with the oil, season with salt and freshly ground black pepper, toss, and spread out on the pan. Roast for about 10 minutes, until browned in spots. Add the corn, mix with the beans, and push to one end of the pan. Put the salmon fillets on the other end of the pan. Season the salmon with salt and pepper.

In a small bowl, mix the mayonnaise with 2 tablespoons of the shredded Parmesan. Spread over the salmon. Sprinkle 2 more tablespoons of the Parmesan on top. Roast for 7 to 9 minutes, until the topping is golden at the edges and the salmon is just done.

PER SERVING: 371 calories, 34 g protein, 24 g carbohydrates, 17 g total fat, 3.5 g saturated fat, 4 g dietary fiber, 332 mg sodium

FAST ITALIAN FISH

A thin slice of prosciutto (Italian ham) infuses delicate whitefish with a subtle saltiness, while a dab of pesto adds color and earthy flavor. Fresh zucchini roasts on the same pan for quick cleanup!

2 or 3 small zucchini

1 teaspoon olive oil

Salt

Freshly ground black pepper

4 slices prosciutto

4 (4- to 5-ounce) halibut or cod fillets

8 teaspoons fresh pesto

Preheat the oven to 425°F.

Trim the ends off the zucchini and cut them lengthwise into quarters. Put them on a nonstick baking sheet, drizzle with the oil, and season with salt and freshly ground black pepper. Roast for 5 minutes.

Meanwhile, wrap 1 slice of prosciutto around each halibut or cod fillet. Remove the pan from the oven, flip the zucchini and push to one side, and put the fish on the pan. Roast for about 8 minutes, until the fish is just opaque and the zucchini are tender. Top each fillet with a little pesto.

PER SERVING: 233 calories, 31 g protein, 4 g carbohydrates, 10 g total fat, 2.5 g saturated fat, 1 g dietary fiber, 814 mg sodium

VEGETABLE PAELLA

MAKES 6 SERVINGS

This versatile Spanish rice dish makes a yummy one-pot meal. It makes a terrific vegetarian dish. Use any short- or long-grain rice. A stubby Spanish variety is traditional—it's similar to the Italian arborio rice available in most supermarkets. This fragrant veggie-rice combo comes together easily. Don't be put off by what looks like a lengthy list of ingredients. More than half of them are pantry and refrigerator staples.

3 tablespoons olive oil

½ red onion, chopped

½ green bell pepper, chopped

12 ounces mushrooms, sliced

2 cloves garlic, minced

1 teaspoon paprika

1 teaspoon dried oregano

1 teaspoon dried thyme

¼ teaspoon freshly ground black pepper

⅛ teaspoon ground red pepper

1½ cups uncooked short- or long-grain rice

2½ cups chicken or vegetable broth (We used Kitchen Basics.)

1½ cups chopped tomatoes (from a 26-ounce box)

1½ teaspoons salt

9 ounces baby spinach, roughly chopped

1 cup frozen peas

1 cup frozen artichoke hearts (halves and quarters)

2 tablespoons red wine vinegar

¼ cup chopped fresh parsley

In a paella pan or Dutch oven, heat the oil over medium heat. Add the onion and cook for 5 minutes, until softened. Add the bell pepper and mushrooms, season with salt to taste, and cook for 3 or 4 minutes, stirring, until softened. Stir in the garlic, paprika, oregano, thyme, and black and red pepper and cook for 1 minute.

Add the rice and then the broth, tomatoes (with juice), and salt. Bring to a boil, reduce the heat, cover, and cook for 15 minutes.

Stir in the spinach, peas, artichokes, vinegar, and 2 tablespoons of the parsley. Season to taste with salt and black pepper. Cover and cook for 5 minutes longer. Remove from the heat and let stand, covered, for 5 minutes. Serve sprinkled with the remaining 2 tablespoons of parsley.

PER SERVING: 358 calories, 13 g protein, 60 g carbohydrates, 9 g total fat, 1.5 g saturated fat, 7 g dietary fiber, 878 mg sodium

DESSERTS

TRIPLE CHOCOLATE CHEESECAKE

MAKES 16 SERVINGS

A mixture of reduced-fat and fat-free cream cheese creates melt-in-your-mouth texture without saturated fat overload.

1 package (9 ounces) chocolate wafer cookies

¼ cup 50-50 butter blend spread, melted

7 ounces semisweet chocolate chips (about 1⅓ cups)

2 packages (8 ounces each) fat-free cream cheese, at room temperature

1 package (8 ounces) reduced-fat cream cheese (Neufchâtel), at room temperature

¾ cup sugar

¼ cup unsweetened cocoa powder

1½ teaspoons vanilla extract

½ teaspoon salt

3 large eggs, at room temperature

Preheat the oven to 325°F. Coat a nonstick 9" springform pan with cooking spray. Set it on a sheet of heavy-duty foil, wrapped up the sides.

In a food processor, grind the wafers to fine crumbs. Set aside ¼ cup. With the processor running, add the spread. Press onto the bottom of the prepared pan. Bake until set, about 12 minutes.

Boil a kettle of water. Melt the chips in the microwave according to the package directions.

Beat the cheeses with an electric mixer on medium speed. Add the sugar, cocoa, vanilla extract, and salt. Beat until fluffy. Add the eggs, one at a time. Beat in the chocolate. Pour the chocolate mixture over the crust. Set in a roasting pan, place in the oven, and pour boiling water between the two pans to reach halfway up the sides of the cheese-cake pan. Bake for about 40 minutes, until the center is almost set but still a bit jiggly.

Crack the oven door open with the handle of a wooden spoon. Turn off the oven and leave the cake in it for 1 hour. Remove from the oven, take the cake from the water, and cool. Remove the foil. Run a knife around the edge of the cake and chill for at least 8 hours. Sprinkle the reserved cookie crumbs on top. Detach the pan sides and smooth the sides of the cheesecake with a knife.

PER SERVING: 272 calories, 9 g protein, 32 g carbohydrates, 14 g total fat, 7 g saturated fat, 2 g dietary fiber, 391 mg sodium.

CARROT CAKE
WITH CREAM CHEESE FROSTING

MAKES 16 SERVINGS

At nearly 600 calories a slice, traditional carrot cake needed some help. We reduced the oil, added applesauce for moisture, and took down the sugar. The perfect amount of sweet and creamy frosting complements the delectable spiced cake.

1½ cups dark brown sugar

¾ cup canola oil

⅓ cup unsweetened applesauce

4 egg whites

2 cups all-purpose flour

2 teaspoons baking soda

2 teaspoons ground cinnamon

½ teaspoon salt

⅛ teaspoon ground nutmeg

⅛ teaspoon ground ginger

2½ cups grated carrots (about ¾ pound carrots)

⅓ cup chopped walnuts

1 cup confectioners' sugar

12 ounces reduced-fat cream cheese (Neufchâtel), at room temperature

½ teaspoon vanilla extract

Preheat the oven to 350°F. Grease and flour a 10-cup Bundt or tube pan.

To make the cake, in a large bowl, combine the brown sugar, oil, applesauce, and egg whites and stir to blend.

In a separate bowl, mix together the flour, baking soda, cinnamon, salt, nutmeg, and ginger.

Beat the dry ingredients into the wet ingredients until smooth. Add the carrots and walnuts and mix until well combined. Pour the batter into the prepared pan and bake for 45 to 50 minutes, until a wooden pick inserted into the cake comes out clean. Allow to cool completely in the pan. Place a rack on top of the pan and invert it to release the cake.

To prepare the frosting, using an electric mixer, gradually beat the confectioners' sugar into the cream cheese and vanilla extract. Spread the frosting on the cooled cake.

PER SERVING: 345 calories, 5 g protein, 44 g carbohydrates, 18 g total fat, 4 g saturated fat, 1 g dietary fiber, 350 mg sodium

LEMON SQUARES

We cut way back on the butter and sugar, with palate-pleasing results. The topping abounds with fresh lemon flavor, while the crust has the sweet, rich taste of shortbread without a lot of calories or saturated fat. Our recipe has 28 percent fewer calories, 43 percent less saturated fat, and 23 percent less sugar than a traditional recipe.

1 cup + 3 tablespoons all-purpose flour

¾ cup granulated sugar

⅛ teaspoon salt

¼ cup butter

1 large egg

1 large egg white

1 large lemon

⅛ teaspoon baking powder

1 teaspoon confectioners' sugar

Preheat the oven to 350°F. Coat an 8" × 8" baking pan with cooking spray.

In a medium bowl, mix 1 cup of the flour, ¼ cup of the granulated sugar, and the salt until well combined. Cut the butter into the flour mixture with a pastry blender until a crumbly dough forms.

Press the dough evenly into the bottom of the prepared baking pan. Bake for 10 to 12 minutes, until lightly golden. Cool.

In a large bowl, whisk the egg, egg white, and remaining ½ cup sugar until combined. Grate and squeeze the lemon and add the peel and juice to the egg mixture. Add the baking powder and the remaining 3 tablespoons flour. Mix thoroughly.

Pour the lemon mixture over the cooled short-bread base. Bake for 20 to 25 minutes, until set and lightly brown at edges.

Cool and dust lightly with the confectioners' sugar using a mesh strainer. Cut into squares.

PER SERVING: 103 calories, 2 g protein, 17 g carbohydrates, 4 g total fat, 2 g saturated fat, 0.5 g dietary fiber, 50 mg sodium

FROZEN STRAWBERRY PIE

MAKES 8 SERVINGS

Loaded with sweet berries, this luscious pie doesn't need full-fat cream cheese to taste delicious. The buttery cookie-crumb crust saves calories over regular pastry. You can make and freeze the pie up to 2 weeks ahead. Just defrost it at room temperature for 35 minutes before serving.

6½ ounces vanilla wafers (about 3 cups)

2 tablespoons butter, melted

2 tablespoons canola oil

8 ounces reduced-fat cream cheese (Neufchâtel), at room temperature

½ cup confectioners' sugar

1 pound strawberries, hulled

1 tablespoon granulated sugar

To make the crust, in a food processor, crush the wafers to fine crumbs. Mix the crumbs, butter, and oil together until combined.

Pack the crumbs on the sides and bottom of a 9" pie plate. Chill the crust for at least 20 minutes or up to a week.

Preheat the oven to 325°F.

Bake the crust for 15 to 18 minutes, until golden. Cool completely.

To prepare the filling, using an electric mixer on medium speed, beat the cream cheese until smooth. Add the confectioners' sugar at low speed. Beat thoroughly at medium speed to combine.

In the food processor, puree one-quarter of the strawberries. Fold the puree (about ⅓ cup) into the filling, saving any extra puree for topping. Pour the filling into the crust. (It will not reach the top.)

Freeze the pie until just firm, about 1½ hours.

To make the topping, quarter or halve the remaining berries. In a medium bowl, toss with the granulated sugar. Let stand for at least 5 minutes. Serve the topping over slices of the pie.

PER SERVING: 283 calories, 4 g protein, 31 g carbohydrates, 17 g total fat, 7 g saturated fat, 2 g dietary fiber, 206 mg sodium

MAPLE-ROASTED PINEAPPLE

MAKES 4 SERVINGS

8 thick slices pineapple

¼ cup pure maple syrup

¼ cup graham cracker crumbs

1 pint low-fat, slow-churned vanilla ice cream

Preheat the oven to 400°F. Coat a baking sheet with cooking spray.

Put the pineapple on the pan, drizzle with the syrup, sprinkle with the crumbs, and coat with cooking spray. Roast for 15 minutes and remove from the oven.

Turn on the broiler. Brush the pineapple with any dripped-off syrup and place under the broiler about 5" from the heat. Broil for 2 to 5 minutes, until charred in spots. Serve warm with the ice cream.

PER SERVING: 258 calories, 4 g protein, 54 g carbohydrates, 4 g total fat, 2 g saturated fat, 3 g dietary fiber, 80 mg sodium

SUPERFOOD: PINEAPPLE

Luscious, tart-sweet pineapple is full of nutrients as well as flavor. Just 1 cup of pineapple offers 37 percent of the daily recommendation for vitamin C.

In addition to supplying vitamin C, a cup contains your daily quota of manganese, a trace mineral that promotes bone health. Though available all year round, this tropical fruit is at its peak from March through June. Go ahead and cut it into chunks and store in the fridge or buy it precut for convenience—the fruit retains its nutritional punch for up to a week.

SPICED GRAPEFRUIT WITH MANGO SORBET

MAKES 4 SERVINGS

½ cup water

¼ cup brown sugar

½ teaspoon ground ginger

2 large grapefruits, cut into segments

4 small scoops mango sorbet

Mint sprigs (optional)

In a small heavy saucepan, simmer the water, sugar, and ginger for about 5 minutes, until reduced to ¼ cup.

Divide the grapefruit sections among 4 dessert dishes. Pour the spiced syrup over the grapefruit, dividing evenly. Top each portion with a scoop of mango sorbet and garnish with a mint sprig (if using).

PER SERVING: 226 calories, 1 g protein, 64 g carbohydrates, 0 g total fat, 0 g saturated fat, 2 g dietary fiber, 15 mg sodium

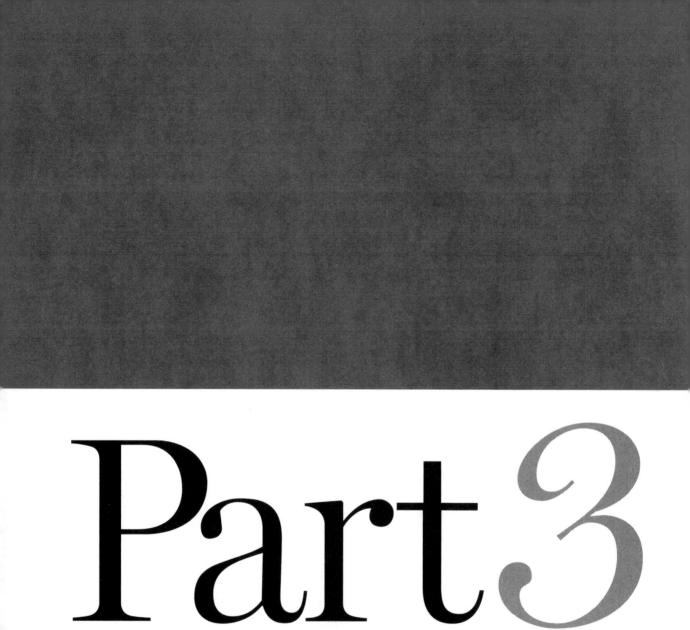

Part 3

FITNESS
MOVES

CHAPTER 12

Faster Toning

Here's the best dumbbell workout to drop pounds, flatten your belly, and firm up your trouble zones

Ask five different personal trainers for the best way to firm up, and you'll likely get five different answers. Though researchers have been investigating weight-lifting techniques for nearly as long as dumbbells have been around, strength training is not an exact science, and many of the studies have been done on college-age guys.

So we decided to find out for ourselves which technique delivers the fastest results, particularly for busy women. We recruited 23 readers, ages 37 to 57, to do six different workouts using dumbbells—the most popular strength-training tool. They all did the same basic exercises (see page 158) but varied the order, amount of weight lifted, and/or number of sets and repetitions; for example, doing circuits with no resting between exercises, traditional training (three sets of 10 to 12 repetitions), or fewer reps with superheavy weights.

And the winner is: drop sets! This technique calls for only two sets of each exercise, without any rest periods. The women in this group lost an average of

5 pounds of fat in just 4 weeks, shrunk their waistlines twice as much as the other groups, and gained enough lean muscle tissue to boost their metabolism by 6 to 9 percent. Even better, it was the speediest routine in the pack, taking just 20 to 25 minutes a session—half the time of some of the other workouts. Drop sets might be so effective because they fatigue muscles—the key to fast results—without making you lift the heaviest weight possible.

According to research, many women choose weights that aren't heavy enough to accomplish this goal. Try the winning workout yourself to tone up and rev your metabolism in half the time of traditional workouts.

PROGRAM AT A GLANCE

What you need: Two or three sets of dumbbells: light (3 to 5 pounds), medium (5 to 10 pounds), and heavy (10+ pounds). Our testers used the Reebok Speed Pac, dumbbells that adjust by $2\frac{1}{2}$-pound increments from $2\frac{1}{2}$ to $12\frac{1}{2}$ pounds, making it easy to progress as you get stronger. (Target and www.target.com; $69.99)

Three days a week: Do the workout that follows on nonconsecutive days, so muscles have time to recover.

Four days a week: Do 30 to 40 minutes of cardio, such as brisk walking, jogging, stationary cycling, swimming, or even dancing. Exercise at an intensity at which you're breathing hard and can only talk in short sentences.

	A: SHORTER DAILY WORKOUTS	B: FEWER BUT LONGER WORKOUTS	C: COMBO PLAN
MON	Strength	Strength & Cardio	Strength & Cardio
TUE	Cardio	Rest	Rest
WED	Cardio	Cardio	Cardio
THU	Strength	Strength & Cardio	Strength & Cardio
FRI	Cardio	Rest	Rest
SAT	Strength	Strength & Cardio	Strength
SUN	Cardio	Rest	Cardio

WAYS EXERCISE SENDS HEALTH SOARING

Whether you're a longtime fitness buff or have recently adopted a more active lifestyle, you reap these rewards every time you lace up.

LIVE LONGER. Vigorous exercisers have longer telomeres—cellular biomarkers that shorten as we age—compared with healthy adults who rarely work out.

TAKE YEARS OFF YOUR BRAIN. Exercise is linked to a lower risk of Alzheimer's disease among older people. Now, new research shows it can prevent brain fog at a much younger age, too. Japanese researchers assigned sedentary young adults to two groups; one took aerobic exercise classes, and the other did not. After 4 months, MRIs revealed that the nonexercising group experienced shrinkage of gray matter in some areas of the brain, while the active participants had no change.

REDUCE INFLAMMATION. Sedentary, obese women age 50 and older who began exercising lowered their levels of C-reactive protein—an inflammatory blood marker linked to heart disease—by 10 percent after 1 year, found research recently published in *Medicine & Science in Sports & Exercise*.

SURVIVE BREAST CANCER. Exercise reduces breast cancer risk, and it can also save your life if you're diagnosed. Overweight women who were exercising more than 3 hours a week before they were diagnosed were 47 percent less likely to die than those who exercised less than ½ hour per week.

FIGHT CIGARETTE CRAVINGS. In a recent *Addiction* study, researchers found that regular smokers were less interested in images of other people smoking after they rode an exercise bike for 15 minutes, compared with when they did not exercise.

Every day: To maximize results, watch portions and fill up on whole grains, vegetables, fruits, lean protein, and healthy fats. Aim for 1,600 to 1,800 calories spread out evenly throughout the day. For calorie-counting help, try our online diet log at www.prevention.com/healthtracker.

Sample schedules: You can configure your workouts to best fit your personal schedule. Here are a few examples.

THE WORKOUT

To do the exercises as drop sets, start with a weight that you can lift for only 10 to 12 reps. Then immediately drop down to the next-lightest weight and complete as many reps as possible. If you can do more than 12, you need to use a heavier weight for the first set. It's okay if you can't do 10; you will as you get stronger. Then go straight to the next move, without resting.

How much weight you use depends on how strong you are to start off with. We've provided a ballpark guide—light, medium, and heavy—for each move. Adjust according to your needs so the final two or three reps are really challenging.

THE EXPERT

Sports physiologist and former Olympic coach Tim Pelot, CSCS, of Pelot Performance Coaching in Burnsville, Minnesota, developed the workout.

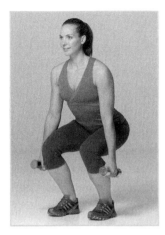

Heavy

ⓒ SQUAT

TONES GLUTES AND THIGHS

Stand tall with your feet hip-width apart, holding dumbbells down at your sides, with your palms facing in. Shift your body weight back into your heels, bend your hips and then knees, and lower, sticking your butt out as if you were sitting in a chair. Keep your head up, shoulders back, abs tight, and back straight as you lower until your thighs are almost parallel with the floor. Make sure that your knees stay behind your toes. (If you look down, you should be able to see your toes.) Pause, then straighten your legs and stand back up.

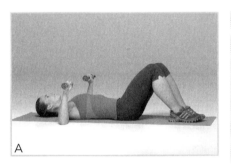

A

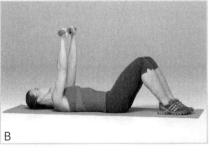

B

Medium to heavy

ⓒ CHEST PRESS

TONES CHEST AND TRICEPS

Holding dumbbells, lie faceup on the floor (or a bench), with your knees bent and your feet flat. Position the weights on either side of your chest with your elbows bent and pointing out to the sides and your palms facing your legs (A). Push the weights straight up over your chest (B). Pause, then slowly lower.

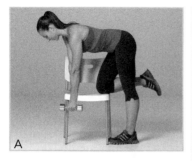

A

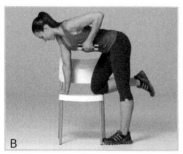

B

Medium to heavy

⊘ BENT-OVER ROW

TONES MIDBACK AND BICEPS

Grasp a dumbbell with your left hand and place your right knee and right hand on a chair (or on a bench) so that your back is parallel with the floor. Keep your head in line with your spine and your abs tight. Let your left arm hang straight down, with your palm facing the chair (A). Bend your left elbow toward the ceiling and pull the dumbbell up toward your chest (B). Pause, then slowly lower. Complete a full set, then repeat with your right arm.

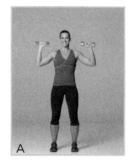

A

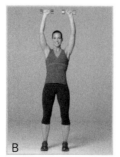

B

Light to medium

⊘ OVERHEAD PRESS

TONES SHOULDERS AND TRICEPS

Stand with your feet hip-width apart. Bend your arms so the dumbbells are just above your shoulders, with your palms facing forward (A). Press the dumbbells straight up overhead, without arching your back (B). Pause, then slowly lower to shoulder height.

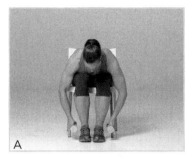

A

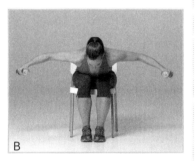

B

Light to medium

⊘ REVERSE FLY

TONES UPPER BACK

Sit on the edge of a chair, with your feet together and a dumbbell in each hand. Lean forward from your hips so your arms hang down next to your calves, with your elbows bent slightly and your palms facing each other (A). Squeeze your shoulder blades together and raise the weights out to the sides, forming an arc, until your arms are about parallel with the floor (B). Keep your elbows slightly bent throughout. Pause, then slowly lower.

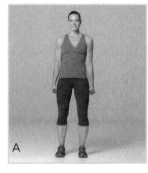

A

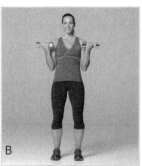

B

Medium

⊘ BICEPS CURL

TONES FRONT OF UPPER ARMS

Stand with your feet hip-width apart. Hold dumbbells at your sides, with your palms facing in (A). Keeping your elbows at your sides, bend your arms, rotate your wrists so your palms face you, and raise the dumbbells up toward your shoulders (B). Pause, then slowly lower.

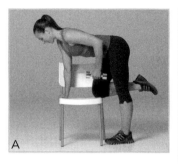

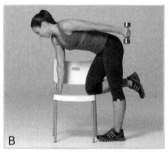

A

B

Light to medium

ⓒ TRICEPS PRESS-BACK

TONES BACK OF ARMS

Hold a dumbbell in your left hand and place your right knee and right hand on a chair (or on a bench) so that your back is parallel with the floor. Bend your left arm so your elbow is at your side and your forearm is perpendicular to the floor (A). Straighten your left arm, raising the weight back toward your butt (B). Pause and slowly return to the starting position. Complete a full set, then repeat with your right arm.

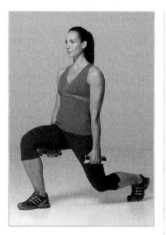

Heavy

ⓒ LUNGE

TONES GLUTES AND THIGHS

Hold dumbbells down at your sides, with your palms facing in. Stand with your right foot 2 to 3 feet in front of your left, with your toes pointing forward, and your left heel off the floor. Bend both of your knees, slowly lowering your left knee toward the floor. Keep your right knee over your ankle; don't lean forward. Pause, then press into your front foot and straighten your legs to stand back up. Complete a full set, then switch legs and repeat.

MIND OVER MIDSECTION

It's true that you might not be able to think yourself thin, but studies suggest that focus and imagination may boost the proven power of diet and exercise. Here's how to make it work for you.

KEEP YOUR EYES ON THE FRIES. People who ate lunch while playing a computer game felt less full than those who dined without distractions, according to a new study from the University of Bristol in England.

CONTEMPLATE THE POSSIBILITIES. Study subjects ate less cheese after they first visualized themselves eating the treat for 1½ minutes, according to scientists at Carnegie Mellon University. Repeatedly imagining the experience diminishes the craving for that food, the researchers speculate.

STAGE A PHOTO FINISH. Want a cupcake? Snap a photo first. Tracking your calories can be a potent way of reminding yourself just how much you're eating. But dieters who photographed everything they consumed were able to reflect on what they were going to eat and make healthier choices, reports a study from the University of Wisconsin-Madison.

CHAPTER 13

New, Simple Ways to Walk Off Weight Three Times Faster

This is no ordinary walking workout. Our reader-tested program powers off pounds, flattens your belly, and firms every inch. Drop a size this month—without dieting!

As a fitness instructor and editor of 20 years at America's leading healthy lifestyle magazine, Michele Stanten walked and talked with hundreds of people at marathons across the country, during test panels for the magazine, and in local neighborhoods and parks. What's the most common walking complaint she heard? "I'm not losing any weight!" That's why she created the Walk Off Weight (WOW) program, based on the latest exercise science, to get you moving, maximize fat loss, and leave lost pounds in the dust for good!

WE TESTED IT!

"I lost 3 inches off my waist in 4 weeks!"—Meg Kranzley, 51

With a fitter body, Meg is unstoppable. She unpacked the entire car, lugging groceries and suitcases, all by herself during a recent vacation. "I didn't feel winded or frazzled," says Meg, who lost 9½ pounds in 4 weeks on the WOW diet and exercise plans.

"I lost over 11 pounds in a month!"—Susan Moyer, 52

This former athlete also strengthened her legs enough to avoid knee surgery for an old injury and has loads of energy. "I went dancing for the first time in years, and I was fit enough to do it all night long," says Susan, who did both the WOW diet and exercise plan.

"I got a better workout in less time!"—Geri Krempa, 46

"By day 14, I felt like a new person," says Geri, who used to take hour long walks. Even her husband commented that her face looked slimmer. "My belly bloat was gone, too!" says Geri, who lost 8 pounds in 4 weeks on the WOW diet and exercise plans.

"I walked a half-marathon!"—Yvonne Shorb, 62

And she completed the 13.1 miles faster than her younger friends who joined her. "I can run after my grandkids, and I biked 33 miles one day," says Yvonne, who lost nearly 7 pounds in 4 weeks following the WOW workouts only. "I feel 20 years younger!"

It's guaranteed to work: Ask the nearly two dozen women, ages 34 to 63, who walked in heat and rain to test this revolutionary program. They lost up to three times the weight that they would have through traditional, steady-paced walking—shedding up to 14 pounds and trimming 3 inches off their waists in just 4 weeks.

The WOW program is designed to keep you out of a walking rut and off those dreaded weight-loss plateaus. The first step is fat-blasting interval walks, in which you'll stride fast for a short period, then slow down to recover before cranking it back up. You'll also do toning walks with an exercise band to firm your upper body while you walk; strength workouts to rev your metabolism; and longer, steady-pace walks to burn more fat.

WORKOUT SCHEDULE

Start the following program today and you could lose as much as 14 pounds, shrink your waist by 3 inches, and drop a size or more in just 4 weeks!

WEEK	DAY 1	DAY 2	DAY 3	DAY 4	DAY 5	DAY 6	DAY 7
1 and 2	30-Minute Interval Walk + Lower-Body Strength Moves 45 minutes total	Toning Walk 20 minutes total	30-Minute Interval Walk + Core Strength Moves 45 minutes total	Toning Walk 20 minutes total	30-Minute Interval Walk + Lower-Body Strength Moves 45 minutes total	Long Walk* + Core Strength Moves 60–75 minutes total	Rest
3 and 4	45-Minute Interval Walk + Lower-Body Strength Moves 60 minutes total	Toning Walk 25 minutes total	45-Minute Interval Walk + Core Strength Moves 60 minutes total	Toning Walk 25 minutes total	45-Minute Interval Walk + Lower-Body Strength Moves 60 minutes total	Long Walk* + Core Strength Moves 90–105 minutes total	Rest

*See page 174 for duration.

PROGRAM AT A GLANCE

What you'll need: Well-fitting walking shoes, a sports watch with interval timer, and a medium-weight elastic resistance band or tube (available at sporting goods stores or online)

What you'll do: A combination of walking and strength workouts (see chart above) 6 days a week

To maximize results: Eat about 1,600 calories a day, filling up on whole grains, fruits, vegetables, lean proteins, and healthy monounsaturated fats. Also have 3 cups of green tea (hot or cold) daily. Studies show compounds in the tea can help you burn belly fat!

WE TESTED THEM! TONING SHOES

Can rounded-bottom "rocker" shoes allow you to walk your way to beautifully sculpted legs—without a single squat? Alas, no. The half-dozen experts we surveyed said you can expect "modest" results, and the risks of injury are real. Here's how to reap the potential benefits. (Skip the sneaks if you have foot, knee, or balance problems.)

BUILD SLOWLY. Some brands are heavier than regular sneakers, so you might fatigue more quickly and walk less. Start with 30 minutes or less and work up to several hours.

CROSS-TRAIN. Once acclimated, wear rockers for shorter, moderate-paced walks on smooth, level surfaces. For longer or fast-paced workouts, use traditional walking shoes.

WEAR FOR A STRENGTH ROUTINE. The balance challenge will firm more muscles in your core and legs. For example, do a yoga bridge pose with your butt lifted, then slowly rock from heels to toes and back.

TONING WALKS

The toning moves that follow are easy to do while you walk. Do twice a week.

Weeks 1 and 2: After you warm up, continue walking at a moderate pace as you do the first exercise for 45 seconds, or about 20 reps. When you're finished, drape the band around your neck and speed up to a brisk pace, as if you're in a hurry, for 1 minute. Repeat the 45-second toning/1-minute brisk walking intervals until you've done all the exercises. Finish with 4 minutes of easy walking to cool down, for a 20-minute routine.

Weeks 3 and 4: Increase the workout to 25 minutes by doing each toning move as you walk for 1 minute, or about 30 reps.

Make it harder: Move your hands closer together so you're using less band.

Make it easier: Separate your hands farther apart so the band is more slack.

PULL-DOWN

FIRMS UPPER AND MIDBACK

Hold the center of the band overhead, with your hands shoulder-width apart, your palms forward, and your elbows bent slightly. Keeping your left hand stationary, pull your right arm down and out to the side to shoulder height, without bending your elbow. Hold, then slowly return to the starting position. (Work your left arm on the next toning interval, after doing a 1-minute brisk walk between moves.)

FRONT PRESS

FIRMS CHEST

Loop the band around your back under your arms. Grasp each side of the band with your hands near your chest, with your palms forward and your elbows pointing out. Extend your arms straight in front of you at chest level. Hold, then slowly return to the starting position.

ROW

FIRMS MIDBACK

Hold the center of the band with both of your hands, with your arms extended in front of you at chest level. Keeping your left arm stationary, bend your right elbow and pull your hand back toward your hip, with your elbow pointing behind you. Hold, then slowly return to the starting position. (Work your left arm on the next toning interval, after a 1-minute brisk walk.)

OVERHEAD PRESS

FIRMS SHOULDERS

Loop the band around your upper back and under your arms. Grasp an end in each hand, with your elbows bent and pointing diagonally down, your hands near your shoulders, and your palms forward. Press your hands straight up overhead. Hold, then slowly return to the starting position.

ARM PULL

FIRMS TRICEPS

Drape the band around your neck. Grasp each side of the band with your arms bent, your hands by your shoulders. Keeping your upper arms stationary, press your hands down and straighten your arms. Hold, then slowly return to the starting position.

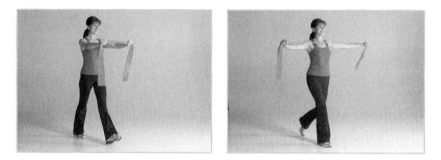

⊼ FRONT PULL

FIRMS UPPER BACK

Hold the band out in front, with your arms extended at chest height and your hands about shoulder-width apart. Keeping your arms straight, pull your hands apart, squeezing your shoulder blades and bringing your hands almost directly out to your sides. Hold, then slowly return to the starting position.

GET FASTER RESULTS!

This program was adapted from *Walk Off Weight* by Michele Stanten (Rodale, 2010). For the complete 8-week Walk Off Weight diet and exercise program, visit www.prevention.com/shop to purchase the book and audio workouts that will talk you through all of these routines and more.

INTERVAL WALKS

In one study, interval exercisers lost more weight with shorter workouts than women who exercised longer at a steady pace. Do three times a week.

TIME	ACTIVITY	INTENSITY	WHAT IT FEELS LIKE
0:00–5:00	Easy walk (5 min)	3–5	Light effort, rhythmic breathing; you can sing.
5:00–6:00	Moderate walk (1 min)	5–6	Some effort, breathing somewhat hard; can speak in full sentences.
6:00–6:30	Fast walk (30 sec)	7–8	Very hard effort, breathless; can manage only yes/no responses.
6:30–7:30	Moderate walk (1 min)	5–6	(see above)
7:30–25:30	Do minutes 6:00–7:30 13 times*		
25:30–30:00	Cooldown (4 min 30 sec)	5–3	Light effort, rhythmic breathing; you can sing.

*For weeks 3 and 4, do minutes 6:00–7:30 23 times. Then begin your cooldown at 40:30, and finish at 45:00.

LOWER-BODY STRENGTH MOVES

Beyond the toned legs and butt you'll get, the following moves will help you walk about 15 percent faster—that's equivalent to increasing your pace from 3.5 mph to 4 mph and burning about 80 extra calories an hour. Do twice a week after walking.

Weeks 1 and 2: Do 12 to 15 reps of each exercise, repeating on both sides.

Weeks 3 and 4: Do 2 sets of 12 to 15 reps of each exercise, repeating on both sides.

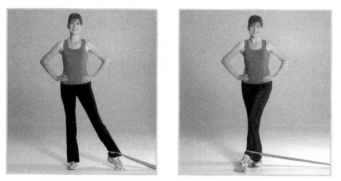

⌃ CROSS LEG SWING

TARGETS INNER THIGHS

Tie the band around a sturdy furniture leg or railing at floor level and loop it around your left ankle (the anchor point is on the left), with your left leg extended out to the side. The band should be taut. Flex your left foot, contract your inner thigh, and swing your left leg across your body. Hold, then slowly return to the starting position without touching your foot to the floor between reps.

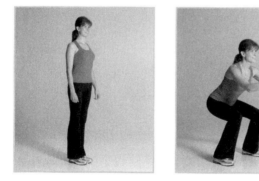

⌃ MOVING SQUAT

TARGETS QUADS AND OUTER THIGHS

Stand with your feet together. Step your right foot out to the side 2 to 3 feet, bend your hips and knees, and sit back as if lowering into a chair. Keep your knees behind your toes. Stand up, bringing your left foot toward your right so your feet are together. Step to the left on the next rep. Alternate sides until you've completed all reps.

CORE STRENGTH MOVES

Strengthening your abs and back will protect you from injury, power your stride so you can go faster—and, of course, flatten your belly! Do the following exercises twice a week after walking.

Weeks 1 and 2: Do 15 to 20 reps (on each side, when appropriate).

Weeks 3 and 4: Do two sets of 15 to 20 reps (on each side, when appropriate).

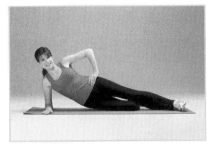 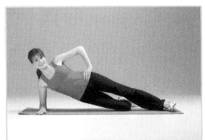

⌃ SIDE PLANK

TARGETS BACK AND ABS

Lie on your right side, with your right leg bent and your left leg extended. Prop yourself up on your right elbow, with your palm flat and your left hand on your hip. Contract your abs and raise your right hip and thigh off of the floor. Slowly lower your right hip without touching the floor in between reps.

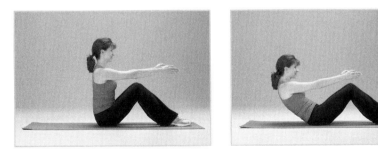

⌃ ROLL-DOWN

TARGETS ABS

Sit on the floor with your knees bent, your feet flat, and your arms extended in front of you. Pull your abs in, round your back, and inhale as you roll about halfway down toward the floor. Exhale and slowly roll up, sitting tall.

LONG WALK

The longer you go, the more calories you'll burn naturally postworkout, research shows. Warm up by walking at an easy pace for about 5 minutes. Increase to a moderate pace for the duration of your walk, finishing with 5 minutes of easy walking to cool down. Do once a week.

WEEK	WALKING TIME*
1	45 minutes
2	60 minutes
3	75 minutes
4	90 minutes

*All times include warmup and cooldown.

BEST NEW EXERCISE SHOES

The latest crop has comfort-enhancing features like lightweight construction and waterproofing, which may be why the 13 avid walkers who wear-tested them easily logged more than 100 miles in about a week. Here are our four favorites.

BEST FOR LONG WALKS: Weighing in at just 9 ounces each, the New Balance 1200 sneakers are light on your feet but as sturdy as heavier shoes.

"They were comfortable and supportive even during the long, hilly walks I take with my dogs," said Stacy Shillinger, 38, Macungie, Pennsylvania. ($120; newbalance.com)

BEST FOR RUNNING INTERVALS: Pick up your pace with Saucony's ProGrid Stabil CS, a running shoe with a reinforced sole that's still flexible enough for walking.

"I felt sure-footed in these shoes, whether I was doing errands or walking for fitness," said Pat Farrell, 45, of Center Valley, Pennsylvania. ($115; saucony.com)

BEST FOR BLISTER PROTECTION: The laces of the Asics Gel-Tech Walker Neo are designed to provide a more secure fit, which can prevent the rubbing that causes blisters.

"The shoe was snug in the heel, but I still had plenty of room in the toe for my feet to spread out," said Mary Lou Phillips, 52, of Germansville, Pennsylvania. ($100; asics.com)

BEST FOR WET OR RUGGED TERRAIN: The Keen Obsidian WP hiker kept feet dry on rainy days, and its thick tread prevented testers from sliding. "These shoes provide heavy-duty protection on trails, but they're as comfortable as a sneaker," said Kathleen Caola, 50, of Bridgewater, New Jersey. ($125; keenfootwear.com)

CHAPTER 14

Our 6-Week Walk-to-Run Program

Yes, you can run! We'll show you how

Running is only for the very fit? Hardly! For decades, scientists have been gathering research that proves running does more good than harm. It doesn't damage knees, and it actually increases your chances of staying active as you get older. It's also effective for weight loss, strong bones, and mental sharpness—at any age! In fact, a new study shows it provides an extra 70 percent reduction in risk of stroke and diabetes—on top of the improvement you'd get from walking for exercise. And people tell us running was the breakthrough that finally busted their weight-loss plateaus. Try our easy plan to safely get you up to speed and running 3 miles straight at any fitness level.

PROGRAM AT A GLANCE

You need: Running shoes to handle the increased impact.

You'll do: Running workouts, alternated with walking and cross-training to work different muscles, condition your body for higher impact and prevent injury.

Three times per week: Run the given distance (see the chart below), taking walking breaks as needed. If you can run only 15 to 30 seconds at a time to start, that's okay. Stop before you're out of breath, walk until you've recovered, and then return to running. Gradually you'll be able to go longer, until, after 6 weeks, you can cover a full 3 miles without walking. (You don't have to be able to run the entire distance to progress each week.)

Once per week: Cross-train. Incorporating different types of workouts helps beat boredom and prevents injury by exercising different muscles. Try swimming to beat the heat and tone your upper body, yoga to stretch and relax your muscles, or cycling to give your legs a break from impact.

Once per week: Walk. This is your easy exercise day, designed to get your blood flowing and loosen up your muscles. Walk at a pace that allows you to chat.

WORKOUT SCHEDULE

	WEEK 1	WEEK 2	WEEK 3	WEEK 4	WEEK 5	WEEK 6
Monday	Run 1.5 miles*	Run 1.75 miles*	Run 2 miles*	Run 2.25 miles*	Run 2.5 miles*	Run 2.75 miles*
Tuesday	Cross-train	Cross-train	Cross-train	Cross-train	Cross-train	Cross-train
Wednesday	Run 1.5 miles*	Run 1.75 miles*	Run 2 miles*	Run 2.25 miles*	Run 2.5 miles*	Run 2.75 miles*
Thursday	Rest	Rest	Rest	Rest	Rest	Walk 30 min
Friday	Run 1.5 miles*	Run 1.75 miles*	Run 2 miles*	Run 2.25 miles*	Run 2.5 miles*	Run 3 miles*
Saturday	Walk 30 to 60 min	Walk 35 to 60 min	Walk 40 to 60 min	Walk 45 to 60 min	Walk 50 to 60 min	Walk 30 to 45 min
Sunday	Rest	Rest	Rest	Rest	Rest	Rest

*Begin and end each workout with 5 minutes of easy walking.

10 FAST FIXES FOR EVERY EXCUSE

Think you have a good reason not to run? Try these simple solutions instead.

My Knees Hurt

Fix #1: Shorten your stride. No matter how cushiony the heel of your shoe is, your body isn't designed to land on it when running, experts say. Shorter strides help you land on the middle of your foot, activating your body's natural shock absorbers.

Fix #2: Strengthen your hips and thighs. One of the most common causes of knee pain is weakness in the thighs and hips, which absorb impact, says runner Alexis Chiang Colvin, MD, an orthopedic surgeon at Mount Sinai School of Medicine. Go to www.prevention.com/knees for targeted toning exercises to keep you pain free.

I Keep Getting Blisters

Fix #3: Check your shoe size. "Your feet increase as much as a size to a size and a half when you run," says running coach and *Runner's World* columnist Hal Higdon. "Especially for new runners, fluids can pool in your extremities, making them swell."

Fix #4: Invest in fancy socks. Yes, there's a difference between $1 and $10 socks. Fabrics that "wick" sweat, including synthetics (like Coolmax) and lightweight wool (like SmartWool), limit friction-causing moisture.

Fix #5: Reduce rubbing. Apply a lubricant such as petroleum jelly or Bodyglide to hot spots before putting your socks on.

It Feels Too Hard

Fix #6: Talk to yourself. Exercisers who repeated an inspiring phrase (such as *I am strong and beautiful!*) aloud at least three times before running a mile went faster and felt better than when they did the same run without the mantra, according to research from the University of Nevada.

Fix #7: Partner up. Not only is exercising with a friend more fun than going solo, but the companionship also may make your workout feel easier, according to a recent British study. Researchers believe the camaraderie may heighten levels of mood-boosting hormones.

I'm Constantly Winded

Fix #8: Slow down. As you become fitter, your body will become more efficient at converting oxygen into energy. Then you'll be able to go faster without getting breathless.

Fix #9: Breathe through your nose and mouth. Forget the old wives' tale that air through your nose is better for you. Quite simply, you need more oxygen to support running or fast walking, and using both your nose and mouth is the most efficient way to get it, says Higdon.

Fix #10: Practice belly breathing. Allowing your chest and belly to expand as you take a breath relaxes your body so it can get oxygen to your muscles more efficiently during exercise, says Susan Joy, MD, director of Women's Sports Health at Cleveland Clinic. Practice it while you're on hold or waiting in line at the grocery store, then try it while you run.

GET MOTIVATED!

Stop watching the clock. It's more efficient (and fun) to track miles instead of minutes. But a treadmill isn't the only way to know your distance. Try these top tips.

Drive. Use your car's odometer to map out a loop. Note landmarks along the way so you'll know how far you've gone when you're running.

Find a track. Many towns have a ¼-mile track at a high school or community center. Four laps equal a mile.

Surf first. Plot your course on a Web site like WalkJogRun.net or try preloaded routes (complete with tips on traffic and hills).

Embrace technology. GPS-powered devices, pedometers, apps, and even some cell phones will measure your distance. Check sporting goods and electronics stores to find a device that meets your needs.

WE'RE RUNNING CONVERTS!

Still skeptical about taking up running? These women didn't think it was for them—until they tried it and were wowed by the incredible results.

Running coach and *Runner's World* columnist Hal Higdon, who has coached thousands of novice runners, designed this program.

．．．

"My legs are strong and toned."—Gwen McCurdy, 51, runner for 10 years

"I was a walker but always had a desire to run—I just didn't think I could, till an acquaintance invited me to join her beginners' running group. Ten years later, I run about 6 miles 5 days a week, and I've even done half-marathons. It's helped me easily maintain a healthy weight for years."

Gwen's advice: "Recruit friends to join you. Running is like therapy. My friends and I talk out all our problems on the run, and afterward life always looks better. Plus the workout flies by."

"I have more energy."—Pam Brantley, 48, runner for 1 year

"I was an on-again, off-again exerciser until some friends talked me into running. I thought it would wipe me out, but I feel more energized on days I run. The first time I ran 20 minutes straight on the treadmill, I felt more exhilarated than I had with any other workout I'd tried. I've lost more than 6 pounds and 16 inches—6 of them from my waistline."

Pam's advice: "Focus on small chunks. Think about what you can do—like running to the next telephone pole or mailbox—and then push yourself to add to it over time."

CHAPTER 15

The Immunity-Boosting Workout

Conquer cold and flu—no sweat! You can boost your flu-fighting immunity with this easy— and fun—20-minute tai chi routine

To keep sick days at bay, trade your vitamin C in for a dose of tai chi. It's cheaper, more effective (revving up your body's disease-fighting defenses by as much as 47 percent), and even triples the protection you get from a flu shot.

The secret to tai chi's elixir-like quality, scientists suspect, lies in its slow movements and controlled breathing. Tai chi marshals the power of both to fight germs. It also zaps stress, and if even helps you to sleep better—both of which are key to a healthy immune system.

Get started with tai chi today with our no-sweat 20-minute routine. You don't even need to change your clothes. The more comfortable you are, the better!

PROGRAM AT A GLANCE

What you'll need: A clutter-free area, about 5 square feet. Tai chi can be done barefoot or in flat, flexible shoes; loose or stretchy comfortable clothing is ideal.

What to do: Perform the routine three to seven times a week. From the beginning stance, you'll repeat the sequence for 20 minutes, and then do the final move.

How to do it: Think of tai chi as a graceful, slow dance. Try each move separately, then link them together into one long sequence. You won't alternate sides like you typically do in workouts.

For best results: Don't worry about hand or feet movements being exact. Tai chi is most effective when you're relaxed.

For more: Find a tai chi class at www.worldtaichiday.org, or try the DVD *Element: Tai Chi for Beginners* (www.collagevideo.com).

Bill Douglas, a Kansas-based tai chi instructor and author of *The Complete Idiot's Guide to T'ai Chi and QiGong,* designed this workout.

. . . .

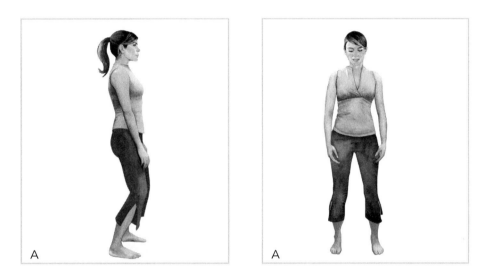

⌃ BEGINNING STANCE

Stand tall with your feet about shoulder-width apart, your toes pointing forward, and your knees bent slightly. Your arms and hands are relaxed at your sides. Look straight ahead and tuck your pelvis slightly to drop your tailbone toward the floor (A). Touch the tip of your tongue to the roof of your mouth to relax your jaw. Inhale through your nose. Pause for a second, and then exhale through your mouth, drawing your navel to your spine. Repeat for three to five breaths. Breathe in this manner as you continue.

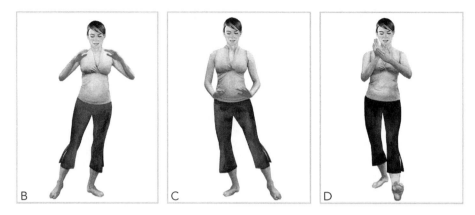

⌃ CIRCLE AND STRIKE PALM

Inhale as you circle your hands up in front of you to chin height, with your palms facing down, and shift your weight to your left leg, bend your left knee slightly, and raise your right heel off of the floor, rotating your foot slightly outward (B). Exhale, lower your hands to about waist height, shift your weight to your right leg, bend your right knee slightly, and raise your left heel (C). Inhale and circle your hands out to your sides. Exhale as your hands come around in front of your chest with your right hand closest to you. Raise your left foot and lightly place your left heel on the floor in front of you, with your foot flexed (D).

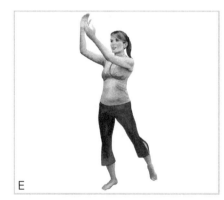
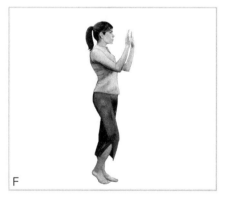

⌃ GRASP AND STROKE BIRD

Inhale, reach both of your hands up diagonally to the right (grasp bird), and tap your left toes on the floor behind you (E). Exhale and swoop your arms down in an arc (stroke bird) as you step your right foot next to your left one, turning your body to face slightly left. Continue circling your hands up until they're in front of your chin, with your palms facing forward (F).

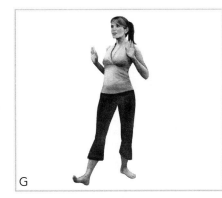

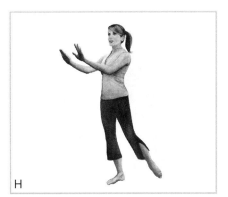

G

H

⌃ PUSHING AND GATHERING ENERGY

Inhale, rotate your torso, and step your right foot to the right, with your foot flexed and your heel touching the floor (G). Exhale and shift your weight onto your right leg (bending the knee slightly) as your left heel comes off the floor and your arms straighten, as if pressing away a heavy object (H).

On the next inhale, step back to the beginning stance (A). Repeat the sequence, moving in the same direction, for 20 minutes. (Even 5 minutes is beneficial if you don't have much time.)

FINAL MOVE

Bring your feet together and inhale as you circle your arms (palms up) out to the sides and overhead. Exhale and slowly lower your hands down in front of your torso, palms down, elbows bent, so your arms end at your sides.

CHAPTER 16

Your Perfect Gym—At Home

Whatever your budget, we'll show you what essentials you need to get a total-body routine under your very own roof. No gym membership required!

No matter if it's too hot outside or too cold, raining, snowing, too windy, anytime is a great time to muzzle some of the most common excuses for not working out—"I'm so busy!" "The weather is so bad!" How? By investing in home exercise gear.

In one study, researchers found that people with home gyms were 73 percent more likely to be active than those without them. Don't worry about knocking down walls, either. You need only one tool to get your heart rate up for a cardio workout and some strength equipment to firm up. We have pinpointed the best options for your budget, along with some extras to help you meet your workout goals.

CARDIO

Choose at least one, and do 30 minutes five or more times a week.

Budget Buys between $20 and $80

Burn 110-plus calories in just 10 minutes with the Reebok Adjustable Speed Jump Rope. You can also add weight to the handles to sculpt shapelier arms. You'll need at least a 9-foot ceiling and a body that can take high-impact exercise. ($20; www.amazon.com)

Another indoor alternative: Step while watching TV, or pop in a DVD for a challenge. Reebok's Incline Step includes slanted risers (for variations that target different muscles) and a 20-minute DVD. ($80; www.amazon.com)

FOUR SNEAKY BELLY FIRMERS

Get toned abs in less time with these twists on traditional moves from Jessica Smith, star of the *10 Minute Solution: Ultimate Bootcamp* DVD.

During Squats

ADD A CHOP: Squat with your arms overhead. As you stand, rotate your torso and quickly swing your arms down toward your hip.

During Pushups

ADD A ROLL: Do a modified pushup on your knees. As you press back up, raise one arm out to side and roll into a side plank.

During Lunges

ADD A CRUNCH: Lunge with your hands behind your head. Hold, then draw your opposite shoulder toward your front knee for an oblique crunch.

During Rows

ADD ROTATION: As you pull a dumbbell up, rotate at the waist so your chest is facing to the side.

HOW TO GET GREAT USED GEAR

Preowned equipment can be a bargain. About 85 percent of home machines sit unused after 18 months, so they're almost like new, says Woody Fisher of Treadmill Doctor, an equipment-servicing outlet. Usage tells more about a machine than its age. Follow our smart-shopping tips for the best deals.

TAKE A TEST DRIVE. Fifteen to 20 minutes is recommended.

GET A WARRANTY. It's usually only available if you're buying through a store.

ASK QUESTIONS. How often was it used? "Mostly as a coat hanger" is code for "buy it now" if everything else checks out. Why are you selling? "I'm trading up for a newer model" means it's probably been used a lot, so pay attention to how smoothly it operates.

LOOK FOR DEAL BREAKERS. Check for an overly dry, cracked, frayed-at-the-edges, or misaligned treadmill belt, as well as any knocks, grinds, high resistance, or excessive friction when any machine is used on a low setting.

DO YOUR RESEARCH. See the used buyer's guide at www.treadmilldoctor.com (look under treadmill or elliptical review tabs). Check with the manufacturer for recalls.

Exercise DVD fans can spice up their routine with Gliding Discs. Stand on them and slide around the room for a low-impact workout that hits underused muscles like the inner thighs. ($23 for discs and 3 DVDs; www.glidingdiscs.com)

Mid-Priced between $599 and $1,000

Pedal off pounds pain free with the Vision Fitness R1500 bike. There's no hunching over handlebars on this recumbent ride, and the cushioned lumbar-supported seat is so comfy, you may not want to get off. ($599; www.visionfitness.com)

Baby your knees and burn megacalories. A no-impact elliptical trainer such as the Nautilus E514 mimics running, and you can reverse directions to work more muscles. This model is so smooth it feels like high-priced gym models. ($999; www.nautilus.com)

FIVE REASONS TO GET OFF THE COUCH!

Here are five new DVDs we love.

Best for Walkers

3 Mile Slim & Sleek Walk

YOU'LL LOVE: The simplicity of three 15-minute indoor walking routines (no treadmill required) that get your heart pumping without any fancy footwork.

BONUS: 12-minute Pilates mat routine

Best Metabolism Blast

3-Week Boot Camp

YOU'LL LOVE: The fat-burning effect of two 20-minute routines that each combine cardio moves and toning with dumbbells into one workout.

BONUS: 6-minute belly-tightening routine

Best Cardio

Barefoot Cardio

YOU'LL LOVE: The invigorating lift you get from this 45-minute blend of Pilates and dance moves that stretches and tones from head to toe.

BONUS: Perfectly paced for beginners, or do in between high-intensity workouts

Best Belly Flattening

10-Minute Solution 5 Day Get Fit Mix

YOU'LL LOVE: The convenience of five quick, effective routines. Do one a day or combine them for longer workouts.

BONUS: A yoga workout to reduce waist-expanding stress

Best Workout That Doesn't Feel Like One

Jazzercise Dancin' Abs

YOU'LL LOVE: The fun you'll have shaking your hips and strutting around your living room during this 60-minute calorie sizzler (or the 30-minute express version).

BONUS: If you're looking for a challenge, the fast-paced choreography delivers.

Fair-weather walkers and runners will like the Horizon Fitness T203 treadmill. Its cushioning system provides more shock absorption at the front of the belt where your foot lands and is firmer at the back where you push off. ($1,000; www.horizonfitness.com)

STRENGTH

Choose at least one product, and do two or three workouts a week.

Budget Buys between $5 and $35

For a high-intensity strength and cardio routine, grab a kettlebell. In just 20 minutes, you can burn up to 400 calories and firm all over. GoFit offers a 10-pound kettlebell with a beginner DVD. ($30; www.gofit.net)

Rubber resistance bands and tubes mimic machine moves and target back, hip, and inner thigh muscles that are hard to hit with dumbbell exercises. Braided Xertubes are a bit pricier but more durable than traditional models. ($30; www.spri.com)

Perfect for beginners, dumbbells are easy to use. Choose lighter ones for small muscles such as triceps, heavier ones for larger muscles. (from about $5 a set; available at retailers such as Sears)

Mid-Priced between $30 and $300

Make body-weight moves such as planks and leg lifts more challenging with Contour-Weights. (You'll probably want two.) Secure the long neoprene tube around your waist, drape it over your leg, or hold it like a bar for upper body exercises. Available in 6, 9, 12, and 15 pounds. ($29 to $55; www.spri.com)

Avoid dumbbell clutter but still challenge yourself with heavy weights (key for fast toning) with Stamina's Versa-Bell weights. You get nine dumbbells in one: A simple click transforms the weight in 2.5-pound increments from 5 to 25 pounds. ($300 per pair; www2.staminaproducts.com)

This portable device is like a gym in a bag. Attach the TRX suspension trainer to a door, put your hands and feet in the handles, and you can do more than 300 exercises. ($190, includes guide and DVD; www.trxtraining.com)

EXCELLENT EXTRAS

For a flatter belly: Exercising on a stability ball activates more ab and back muscles for faster firming. The TrainerBall makes it easy: Moves are printed right on the ball. ($30; www.trainermat.com)

For better balance: Basic moves like stepping forward and back become more challenging on the 6-inch-wide Beamfit Activity Beam. The result is a gentle strength and flexibility workout that targets your core and improves stability. ($125; www.beamfit.com)

For cyclists: Turn your bike into an indoor cardio machine by hooking it up to the CycleOps Magneto bike trainer. It even provides progressive resistance: As you pedal faster, the difficulty increases without your having to shift gears. ($280; www.cycleops.com)

journal

"I'VE NEVER HAD SO MUCH ENERGY"

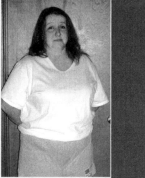

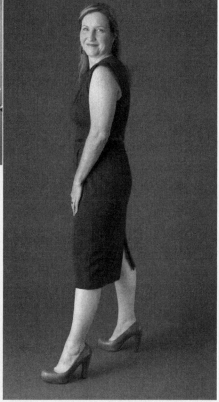

I began eating right and exercising for the sheer joy of it. I'm now a size 6

by Priscilla Bartlett

When I was growing up, the family dinner was meat and potatoes. Though I was never an athletic girl, I was active, and that, combined with my youthful metabolism, kept my weight in check at 120 pounds—until I grew up and got married.

My husband, George, and I continued to eat heavy, high-fat dinners—including takeout fried chicken and pizza accompanied by lots of beer! After 15 years, George had put on 20 pounds, but I'd gained 85.

Worried about my health, George suggested going on a diet together. We decided to replace breakfast and lunch with high-protein shakes. Along with controlling calories, it gave me the structure I needed after years of mindlessly snacking all day on junk. To supplement the shakes, we ate veggie-packed snacks and a sensible dinner.

Still, I knew dieting alone wasn't enough, so I started walking a mile every day. After 3 months, I was covering 3 to 4 miles at a time—and looking for a new challenge. Then one day my husband, who'd cycled since before we got married, surprised me with a new bike.

We soon started riding 15 to 18 miles every weekend and eventually began doing charity rides. The most challenging one was 50 miles. The last 8 miles included lots of hills, which have never been my strong suit. But I found my comfort zone and made it to the finish line.

When I started biking, I'd already lost 59 pounds. After we started cycling regularly, the last 26 pounds flew off! Along the way, I transitioned from meal-replacement shakes to healthy, balanced meals, which helped fuel my exercise.

Today I ride every weekend and two or three times a week. I'm so much happier: I've dropped from size XXL shirts to small/medium. More important, I have lots more energy. I'm no longer ashamed of the way I look, and my husband can't keep his hands off me! He's proud of me, and I'm proud of him for supporting me in such a loving way. I could not have done it without him.

Here are my top tips.

EXERCISE FOR JOY, NOT JUST WEIGHT LOSS. Cycling was an epiphany for me. It gets me outdoors, clears my head, and helps maintain my weight. To stay on track, I also get on the scale every morning.

BE A SOUNDING BOARD. Co-workers often come to me with their frustrations about losing weight. I never judge anyone, because I've been there; I want only the best for them. It also reminds me that wow, I actually did this!

MAKE ROOM FOR FOODS YOU LOVE. When I started dieting, I incorporated chocolate—my weakness—into my new plan.

HAVE A BACKUP ROUTINE. When the weather's bad, I hook up my bike to a stationary indoor bike trainer so I can still get my workout.

RETRAIN YOUR TASTEBUDS. It took a while, but now I look forward to healthy foods such as salad, steamed broccoli, and grilled fish or chicken.

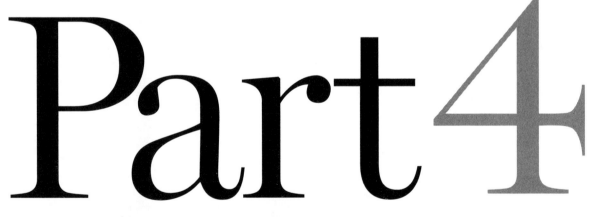

Part 4

NUTRITION
NEWS

CHAPTER 17

The New Power Foods

New research into everyday foods reveals what you should specifically eat to reach any health goal

Blueberries, broccoli, walnuts: You know these superfoods fight disease and boost health. But are they the best choices for your personal health goals? Science suggests it may be time for you to branch out. A recent surge in clinical research reveals a new crop of superfoods that can help lower your risks of everything from cancer and heart disease to macular degeneration and osteoporosis.

For extra motivation (because, of course, you do your best to avoid junk food, too), we've included the latest studies on surprising culprits that make these problems worse. Eat a daily dose of the right foods—and purge your diet of these health saboteurs—to get the health benefits you want most.

PROTECT YOUR HEART
Fill up on these . . .

Barley: This grain can blast LDL ("bad" cholesterol) and triglycerides, lowering your total cholesterol an average of 13 points—without affecting your HDL ("good" cholesterol) levels, according to a 2009 research review. Barley contains beta-glucan, a type of soluble fiber that binds with cholesterol to whisk it from the body, explains David Grotto, RD, the author of *101 Optimal Life Foods*. A cup and a half of cooked pearled barley contains 3 grams of soluble fiber, the daily amount recommended by the FDA.

Pinto beans: Like barley, pinto beans contain cholesterol-fighting beta-glucan. In one study, participants with mild insulin resistance (a precursor to high cholesterol) who ate $1/2$ cup of pinto beans daily dropped 19 points from their total cholesterol level in 8 weeks, including a 13-point decrease in LDL.

Grapes: Consuming just $1\frac{1}{4}$ cups of grapes can prevent the damaging effects of a high-fat meal that can slow circulation and increase risk of coronary heart disease, say researchers at Nationwide Children's Hospital in Columbus, Ohio. A daily dose of grapes improves blood vessel health in general, scientists believe, because the fruit contains high levels of antioxidants called polyphenols.

THE BEST POWER COMBO FOR YOUR BELLY

Sometimes power foods work best in pairs. For example, stave off tummy-aches by stirring some blueberries into your breakfast yogurt. The nutritious fruit boosts yogurt's natural ability to quell inflammation in your gut, Swedish researchers recently found.

The benefits are twofold: The fruit's fiber helps yogurt's "good" probiotic bacteria survive the trek through your digestive tract, where they help boost intestinal health. At the same time, the probiotic bacteria help increase absorption of fiber from the berries.

Macadamia nuts: An Australian study published in the *Journal of Nutrition* found that when men with high cholesterol ate between 1 and 3 ounces of macadamia nuts per day for 1 month, their LDL dropped by 5.3 percent, while their HDL rose by 7.9 percent. The nuts, researchers concluded, increased the amount of healthy monounsaturated fatty acids (MUFAs) in the blood. One ounce is adequate for most people.

Mineral water: The magnesium and calcium plentiful in most mineral waters (such as San Pellegrino, which has 56 milligrams of magnesium and 208 milligrams of calcium) are both potential blood pressure reducers. In a Swedish study, 70 men and women ages 45 to 64 with borderline hypertension experienced a significant decrease in blood pressure after 4 weeks of drinking 1 liter of mineral (not seltzer) water daily.

Avoid these . . .

Energy drinks: The caffeine and guarana that are often added to energy drinks can make your blood pressure skyrocket, says John La Puma, MD, the author of *ChefMD's Big Book of Culinary Medicine.*

STRENGTHEN YOUR BONES
Fill up on these . . .

Lean top sirloin: A 4-ounce serving of this cut (grass or grain fed) provides more than half the Daily Value (8 milligrams) of zinc, a bone-protecting mineral. Research shows that low levels of zinc are associated with brittle bones in middle-aged women. If you prefer seafood, an Alaskan king crab leg packs 10 milligrams.

Broccoli: Broccoli is bursting with vitamin K, which helps your body transport calcium and metabolizes the mineral into your skeleton. Several studies found that vitamin K boosts bone mineral density in osteoporosis sufferers, and it also reduces fracture rates. As a result, the Institute of Medicine upped its daily recommendation to 90 micrograms for women and 120 micrograms for men (3.5 ounces of broccoli contains 141 micrograms). Other good sources include broccoli rabe and spinach.

Avoid this . . .

Salt: Excess sodium increases the amount of calcium excreted in your urine. Over time, this could lead to significant bone loss, say British researchers. Grotto recommends limiting sodium intake to 2,300 milligrams daily.

PROMOTE DIGESTION
Fill up on these . . .

Blueberries: These colorful berries aren't just good for your brain. They contain high concentrations of anthocyanins, which are compounds that can reduce the risk of colorectal cancer by 33 percent, according to a study of more than 6,000 people published in *Cancer Epidemiology, Biomarkers & Prevention*. Grotto recommends eating a daily cup of blueberries—or cherries, strawberries, or Concord grapes, which also contain anthocyanins.

Popcorn: This popular snack is rich in insoluble fiber, which helps keep your digestive system moving. Snacking on 3 cups of air-popped (not microwave) popcorn twice a week can reduce your risk of diverticular disease, a painful inflammation of the intestine, by 28 percent, according to a 2008 study published in the *Journal of the American Medical Association*.

Bananas: Add a banana to your daily morning cereal to get a healthy dose of protease inhibitors, compounds that fight off *H. pylori*, which is the bacterium that researchers believe is the cause of most stomach ulcers.

Avoid these . . .

Dried plums: Although filled with healthy fiber, dried plums are also high in sorbitol, which is a sugar alcohol that in large quantities can cause gas, bloating, and sometimes diarrhea. Grotto suggests limiting your intake to four or five plums a day or substituting a sorbitol-free dried fruit, such as apricots.

SHARPEN YOUR VISION
Fill up on these . . .

Collard greens: People who eat at least two daily servings of leafy greens, such as collard greens and spinach, are 46 percent less likely to develop macular degeneration, which is a leading cause of blindness in those over age 60, according to Harvard Medical School. These foods contain lutein and zeaxanthin, two powerful carotenoids that help eyes absorb short wavelength light and protect the retina, says Dr. La Puma. Women with diets high in beta-carotene (of which collard greens are a rich source) were 39 percent less likely to develop serious cataracts, according to a Harvard Medical School study of more than 50,000 nurses. Because beta-carotene is fat soluble, cook the greens first, then add olive oil to maximize absorption.

Low-fat or fat-free milk: Low-fat and fat-free milk have plenty of riboflavin, which is a B vitamin that helps prevent cataracts. Your body uses riboflavin to manufacture glutathione, which fights free radicals that can damage eye tissue. In addition, vitamin D, found in fortified milk, might protect your eyes. One study showed that people with high blood levels of vitamin D reduced their risk of macular degeneration by nearly 40 percent, compared with people with low levels.

Nuts: The omega-3 fatty acids in nuts, especially walnuts, reduce inflammation and prevent oxidative damage to the retina, says Grotto. Just one or two weekly servings of about ¾ ounce of nuts lower your risk of developing early macular degeneration by 35 percent, according to new research published in the *Archives of Ophthalmology*.

Avoid these . . .

Refined foods: People who regularly eat white bread, cornflakes, and other foods that spike blood sugar almost double their risk of macular degeneration, according to a 10-year Tufts University study of more than 4,000 subjects. Switch to whole grain versions of bread and cereal to steady your blood sugar.

PROTECT YOUR BREASTS
Fill up on these . . .

Cauliflower: This cruciferous vegetable contains sulforaphane, which halted the growth of breast cancer cells in test-tube studies by interfering with the cells' ability to reproduce. Cauliflower also contains a compound called I3C, which may lower levels of estrogens that might otherwise encourage tumors to multiply. When cooking this veggie, roast or steam but never boil it; new research says boiling causes up to 75 percent of the cancer-fighting compounds to leach into the cooking water.

Sweet potatoes: One 5-inch-long sweet potato contains 11,062 micrograms of beta-carotene, a carotenoid that helps your body metabolize estrogen better, says Dr. La Puma. Women with the lowest levels of beta-carotene and other carotenoids had double the risk of breast cancer than those who had the highest levels, found the New York University Women's Health Study.

Tomato sauce: Research shows that lycopene, a powerful antioxidant found in tomato sauce, might protect against breast cancer by neutralizing free radicals that damage cells. Studies prove that lycopene can inhibit breast cancer cell growth in test tubes as well as suppress tumors in mice. Plus, it helps shield skin from cancer-causing sun damage. Lycopene is more easily absorbed in the body when exposed to heat, so cooked tomatoes are better than raw. Lycopene is fat soluble, so add olive oil to help absorption.

Avoid this . . .

Grapefruit: Eating just one-quarter of a grapefruit each day or one-half every other day might increase a postmenopausal woman's chances of developing breast cancer by up to 30 percent, according to a 9-year University of Southern California study of 46,000 postmenopausal women. Although doctors aren't sure exactly why, several studies show that grapefruit interacts with estrogen and increases its potency—so much so that the FDA requires hormone replacement medications to carry a warning label concerning grapefruit juice.

CLEAR YOUR LUNGS
Fill up on these . . .

Pears: These fruits contain quercetin, a powerful flavonoid that might protect the lungs. A Dutch study of more than 13,000 people found that those who ate the most pears (as well as apples, which also contain quercetin) had the best lung function, while an Australian study discovered a strong association between high pear and apple consumption and lower risk of asthma.

Edamame: People with lung cancer tend to have low levels of phytoestrogens, important plant compounds, according to a study in the *Journal of the American Medical Association*. Women who ate the highest quantities of foods containing phytoestrogens, such as edamame, tofu, and lentils, slashed their lung cancer risk by 34 percent.

Brown rice: This grain is high in selenium, which might help keep lung-damaging free radicals from forming. A New Zealand study found that people who got the most selenium were nearly two times less likely to develop asthma than those who got the least. You'll meet the DV of 55 micrograms with a few servings of selenium-rich foods, such as whole wheat bread, chicken, and eggs.

Avoid these . . .

Soft drinks: If you have asthma, skip soft drinks, advises Dr. La Puma. Many contain food additives such as sodium benzoate, MSG, and sulfites, which can exacerbate symptoms.

PAIN PROOF YOUR JOINTS
Fill up on these . . .

Olive oil: Just 2 teaspoons of olive oil (plus 3 grams of fish oil) a day might significantly improve morning stiffness, joint pain, and fatigue, according to a Brazilian study. Research also shows a high intake of olive oil might reduce the risk of rheumatoid arthritis by up to 61 percent.

Oranges: Vitamin C activates a gene that helps cartilage synthesis, says Dr. La Puma. People who eat the most vitamin C–rich foods have 70 percent less cartilage loss than those who don't—and slow the progression of osteoarthritis by 300 percent, according to the Framingham Osteoarthritis Cohort Study.

Avoid this . . .

Beer and hard liquor: If you're prone to gout, avoid beer (just one daily boosts by 15 percent your uric acid levels, high measures of which can cause gout) and hard liquor (which raises it by 12 percent), according to a Harvard Medical School study of more than 14,000 people.

BOOST YOUR MEMORY
Fill up on these . . .

Apples: Eating two or three apples a day increases levels of acetylcholine, a neurotransmitter crucial to maintaining memory that tends to decrease with age, according to research from the University of Massachusetts. Additionally, antioxidants in the fruit protect brain cells from free radical damage.

Chicken breast: In a study of more than 6,000 people conducted by the Rush Institute for Healthy Aging and the CDC, those who ate foods high in niacin, such as chicken breast, yellowfin tuna, and Chinook salmon, had a 70 percent lower risk of mental decline and Alzheimer's disease. Aim for at least 14 milligrams of niacin daily, the amount in 3.5 ounces of roasted skinless chicken breast.

Coffee: People who drank 3 to 5 cups of filtered java a day reduced their risk of dementia and Alzheimer's by 65 percent, according to results from a Finnish/Swedish study of more than 1,400 people over 2 decades by the University of Kuopio and published in the *Journal of Alzheimer's Disease.*

Avoid this . . .

Liver: This meat—along with turnip greens and shiitake mushrooms—has large amounts of copper. A diet high in this mineral (2,750 micrograms daily) is associated with a faster rate of cognitive decline by the equivalent of 19 years, research shows, if you eat it in a diet high in saturated and trans fats.

SMOOTH YOUR SKIN
Fill up on these . . .

Canned light tuna: This kitchen staple is packed with selenium, an antioxidant that protects skin cells against sun damage that can lead to skin cancer. People whose blood had the highest levels of selenium had a 57 percent lower rate of developing basal cell carcinoma and a 64 percent reduction in squamous cell carcinoma, compared with those with the lowest levels, according to a 2009 Australian study of almost 500 adults. Other selenium sources include turkey and fortified instant cereal. The Daily Value for selenium is 55 micrograms, the amount found in a little less than 3 ounces of canned light tuna.

Dark chocolate: New research shows that women who consumed a daily drink containing 2 tablespoons of high-flavonoid cocoa powder for 12 weeks had skin that was significantly smoother, retained more moisture, and had better circulation. Grotto says you can achieve the same effect with a daily ounce of high-flavonoid dark chocolate.

Black tea with citrus peel: Longtime tea drinkers enjoy half the risk of skin cancer—especially if they sip 2 or more cups each day, according to a 2007 Dartmouth Medical School study. That's possibly due to tea's polyphenols, which might help protect against UV radiation. Brew tea with citrus peel to boost its anticancer powers even more. The combined theaflavins in black tea and the d-limonene in citrus reduced the risk of squamous cell carcinoma by 88 percent, says research from a University of Arizona College of Public Health study.

Carrot juice: One cup of carrot juice (which is equal to 1 pound of carrots) contains 22 milligrams of beta-carotene, a powerful antioxidant that several studies show can help protect skin against sunburn. And the more you drink, the more protection you build up.

Avoid this . . .

Alcohol: Scientists aren't exactly sure why, but drinking more than two alcoholic beverages a day raises your risk of basal cell carcinoma by up to 30 percent, according to research at Harvard School of Public Health.

CHAPTER 18

Bonus Antioxidants

Some antioxidants are well known, but others are turning up in surprising places. Where are your antioxidants hiding?

When scientists first discovered the power of antioxidants to destroy cell-damaging free radicals, the hunt was on. They knew these preventers of cancer and heart disease were in colorful fruits and vegetables and nuts, but recently researchers have uncovered them in new, unexpected places.

"The number and variety of these kamikaze substances we find in foods continue to grow," says Christine Gerbstadt, MD, RD, of the American Dietetic Association.

And that's a good thing, experts say, because upping your antioxidant intake from as many sources as possible is more beneficial than getting them from just a few highly publicized foods.

"Don't just eat blueberries every day and think you're covered," says Joe Vinson, PhD, an analytical chemist at the University of Scranton who specializes in measuring antioxidant levels of foods. "When you eat a diverse diet, you get the entire spectrum of benefits they deliver." Here's where they're hiding.

IN YOUR WHOLE GRAIN PASTA

Whole grain versions of pasta (whole wheat should be listed as the first ingredient) have three times more antioxidants than enriched or refined varieties, found Dr. Vinson's study at the University of Scranton. He and his team compared the enriched or refined with the whole grain versions of three spaghetti brands.

"Many epidemiological studies show that the consumption of whole grains can reduce the risk of heart disease," he says. "We used to think this was because of the fiber sweeping out the cholesterol, but it's looking more like it's the polyphenols' positive effect on blood pressure and other markers of heart health that deserve the credit." The concentrations of antioxidants in whole grain flour used to make wheat pasta are comparable to those found in fruits and veggies.

IN YOUR POPCORN

Popcorn has four times more polyphenols—powerful cancer-fighting plant compounds—than the average amount found in fruits, says Dr. Vinson, who tested several whole grain foods to measure antioxidant levels.

"When air-popped at home, it's a 100 percent whole grain food, so it's not a complete surprise that it's packed with polyphenols," he says.

QUICK TIP WE LOVE: POWER UP YOUR PEANUTS

For a bigger antioxidant punch per crunch, roast shelled peanuts at 350°F for 21 minutes. Add to salads or stir-fries. Include the antioxidant-rich seed coats, which might shed during cooking. The heat releases twice as many disease-fighting compounds, such as coumaric acid, which might help combat cancer, say USDA researchers.

278

THE NUMBER OF MILLIGRAMS OF HEART-HEALTHY FLAVONOIDS IN A CUP OF GREEN TEA, ACCORDING TO THE USDA DATABASE FOR THE FLAVONOID CONTENT OF SELECTED FOODS

IN YOUR EGGS

Eggs aren't commonly considered a rich source of the antioxidant lutein (which protects your eyes from macular degeneration and cataracts) because they have low concentrations of it, relative to top sources such as spinach. However, scientists at the Jean Mayer USDA Human Nutrition Research Center on Aging at Tufts University discovered that the lutein in egg yolks is absorbed more effectively than that in spinach, possibly because the yolks' fat helps our bodies process the antioxidant much better.

So even though one egg has only about 5 percent of the lutein found in just ¼ cup of spinach, we absorb it three times more effectively, explains Elizabeth Johnson, PhD, coauthor of the Tufts study. "Spinach and other leafy greens are still the best sources, but whole eggs are another easy way to get more lutein," she says.

IN YOUR CANNED BEANS

A 2004 study conducted by the USDA found that certain varieties of dried beans contain high levels of antioxidants, but Americans more commonly eat canned beans, observes scientist Mark Brick, PhD. To find out if canned have as many antioxidants as dried, Dr. Brick and a team of researchers at Colorado State University measured the phenolic and flavonoid contents of several types of canned commercial beans for a 2009 study published in *Crop Science.*

The scientists found that while all canned beans contain antioxidants, small red beans have the highest levels, followed closely by dark red kidney and black beans. In fact, darker canned beans have as much as three times more phytochemicals—plant compounds that wipe out free radicals to protect your cells and repair DNA damage—than white kidney and great Northern beans.

IN YOUR YOGURT

Love yogurt? You'll love this stat: Just 1 cup of low-fat plain yogurt provides at least 25 percent of the Daily Value for riboflavin—the same that's in 1 cup of boiled spinach. While not an antioxidant itself, riboflavin (a B vitamin) is critical

ADD TO SMOOTHIES. Blend 1 unpeeled kiwifruit, ½ cup frozen strawberries, 1 cup orange juice, and ½ cup plain yogurt.

Orange Peels

They provide d-limonene, a compound that might protect against skin cancer.

ADD TO CHILI. Finely chop the peel and toss in 1 or 2 tablespoons with the beans, tomatoes, and spices.

Broccoli Stalks

A single stalk contains more than a day's worth of vitamin C.

ADD TO STIR-FRIES. Peel the stalks—what's inside is almost as tender as asparagus and makes a delicious addition.

Carrot Peels

The beta-carotene protects the eyes, skin, and immune system.

ADD TO MEAT LOAF AND BURGERS. Mix shredded carrot and carrot peel with lean ground meat to keep it from drying out.

in promoting antioxidant activity. Without it, the antioxidant glutathione—which is already in our cells—cannot destroy free radicals, which might lead to an increased risk of heart disease, cancer, and other chronic conditions. Because riboflavin is water soluble, it remains in the body only a few hours and must be replenished daily. Yogurt does the trick.

IN YOUR CANOLA OIL

Heart-healthy canola oil (which is less expensive and milder tasting than olive oil) is rich in the antioxidant alpha-tocopherol, according to Maret Traber, PhD, of the Linus Pauling Institute at Oregon State University. Just

1 tablespoon contains 16 percent of the DV. Alpha-tocopherol is one of eight antioxidants in vitamin E, which scientists have found keeps the fats in "bad" LDL cholesterol from oxidizing and forming free radicals, potentially leading to cardiovascular diseases and other chronic conditions.

Turns out, though, we aren't getting enough of this potent antioxidant. Close to one-third of women have low concentrations of alpha-tocopherol, say researchers who looked at data from a national nutrition survey conducted by the CDC. Easy fix: Use canola oil when baking or anytime you need a neutral-tasting oil for sautéing.

IN YOUR ORGANIC MILK

Switch from regular milk to organic and you'll be rewarded with a stronger dose of antioxidants, including vitamin E and the carotenoids beta-carotene and lutein, says Gillian Butler, PhD, coauthor of a recent British study published in the *Journal of the Science of Food and Agriculture*.

Dr. Butler's findings show that the antioxidants in milk from cows raised on organic or grass-fed diets are about 40 to 50 percent more concentrated than the milk from conventionally raised cows. These cows eat more grass, and the pasture itself provides more antioxidants than grain feeding even if the feed is augmented with supplements. If you're not a frequent milk drinker, look for cheese and butter from grass-fed cows; they also offer more antioxidants than conventional varieties, says Dr. Butler.

IN YOUR NATURAL SWEETENERS

The average American consumes 130 grams of added refined sugars each day. If you cut excess sugar and use natural sweeteners such as molasses, honey, brown sugar, and maple syrup instead of refined sugar whenever possible, you can add antioxidants equivalent to an extra serving of nuts or berries to your daily diet.

That's according to researchers at Virginia Tech University who examined the antioxidant content of several natural sweeteners and found that molasses

HOT IDEA: EAT YOUR TEA!

How can you reap the heart and brain benefits of tea without drinking the 2 to 5 cups a day that many recent studies suggest? By infusing it into your favorite recipes. Tea can impart a unique flavor to food without adding calories, sodium, sugar, or fat and is one of the best dietary sources of age-erasing antioxidants, says chef Robert Wemischner, coauthor of *Cooking with Tea.* Try one of these supersimple ways to give your family's meals a tasty health boost.

AS A RUB: Grind 1 teaspoon of black tea leaves in a spice mill and add to your favorite spice mixture. Rub onto uncooked chicken, beef, or fish. Let stand 10 minutes before cooking.

Tip: Use loose leaf tea or just tear open a bag.

AS A STOCK: Add brewed tea to broth and pour over meat or fish for braising.

Tip: Use black teas where you would typically add red wine, and green tea or oolong in place of white wine.

AS A MARINADE: Warm 1 teaspoon black tea leaves in 1 cup freshly squeezed orange juice. Remove from the heat and let steep for 5 minutes, then strain and discard the leaves. Refrigerate scallops or shrimp in the mixture for 15 to 60 minutes before cooking.

Tip: To make sauce, add 1 small clove garlic (finely minced) and 1 tablespoon soy sauce and bring to a boil, then simmer until reduced. Spoon over seared scallops.

(particularly dark and blackstrap varieties) had the highest amounts. Their study, published in the *Journal of the American Dietetic Association,* showed that honey, brown sugar, and maple syrup also contained significant levels of antioxidants. While the university study looked at commonly available commercial honeys (usually refined from clover nectar), earlier studies have measured antioxidants in a variety of honeys and found that darker types tend to have significantly higher polyphenol counts. For example, buckwheat has an antioxidant level eight times higher than that of clover, which is also outranked by sunflower and tupelo honeys.

CHAPTER 19

The Case for Natural Foods

There's one change every woman should make this year: Choose real, whole foods over processed, fake ones. Here, nutrition doc David Katz, MD, MPH, tells you why this approach guarantees lifelong health

We are what we eat. We've all heard it, but most of us probably don't quite believe it. After all, you've had french fries and didn't sprout french fry antennae. So we're not really what we eat . . . are we?

We are. It's every bit as true as it is hard to see. Just as our homes are made from lumber without looking like trees, our bodies are made from the nutrients we extract from foods without resembling those foods. The nutritional content of what we eat determines the composition of our cell membranes, bone marrow, blood, and hormones. Consider that the average adult loses roughly 300 billion cells to old age every day and must replace them. Our bodies are literally manufactured out of the food we consume.

That's why what we put in them is of utmost importance—and why "clean food" is an urgent priority and "junk" food is neither cute nor innocuous. In short, our bodies are only as clean as the food we feed them.

What difference does that make? Nothing less than this: Our forks—and our feet—are the master levers of medical destiny. Before 1993, a list of the leading causes of death in the United States included heart disease, cancer, and stroke. But in that year, J. Michael McGinnis, MD, and William Foege, MD, changed this paradigm when they published "Actual Causes of Death in the United States" in the *Journal of the American Medical Association,* which looked at the causes of these diseases.

They concluded that fully half the annual deaths—roughly a million—were premature and could've been postponed by modifying *behaviors,* including smoking, diet and exercise, alcohol consumption, use of firearms, sexual behavior, motor vehicle crashes, and illicit drug use. Smoking and poor eating and exercise habits alone accounted for 700,000 premature deaths in 1990.

In 2004, a group of scientists at the CDC revisited this issue in *JAMA* and came to the same conclusion. This time, however, the toll from bad eating had gone up due to obesity and diabetes.

Then, in 2009, CDC scientists published a paper in the *Archives of Internal Medicine* analyzing records of more than 23,000 German adults enrolled in the European Prospective Investigation into Cancer and Nutrition study (EPIC) and investigated four behaviors: Are you eating well? Are you a healthy weight? Are you physically active? Do you smoke?

People with four good answers (eating well, body mass index below 30, active, not smoking), compared with those with four bad answers (not eating well, BMI above 30, not active, and smoking), were 80 percent less likely to have any major chronic disease. (Imagine if a pill could reduce our risk of dying prematurely from any cause by 80 percent!)

You have doubtless heard of nature (genes) versus nurture (environment), but this shows that lifestyle is so powerful, we can use it to nurture nature, or influence our genes. Various studies have shown this, but Dean Ornish, MD, and his colleagues have produced the most compelling results. Assigning men with prostate cancer to a "clean living" intervention that included a wholesome, plant-based diet; regular physical activity; and stress management, they demonstrated a marked reduction in the activity of genes that can promote prostate cancer growth and a significant increase in the genes that are able to control it.

IT *IS* EASY BEING CLEAN

That's the power and promise in clean eating, so it helps to know what it means. Is it organic? Not necessarily. Food can be organic without being nutritious—think organic gummy bears—or nutritious without being organic, such as conventionally grown broccoli. Organic is a good thing, but it's not a summary measure of "clean."

Clean foods are minimally processed and as direct from nature as possible. They're whole and free of additives, colorings, flavorings, sweeteners, and hormones. Look for foods with one-word ingredients, such as spinach, blueberries, almonds, salmon, and lentils. The longer the ingredient list, the more room there is for manufacturing mischief—additions of chemicals, sugar, salt, harmful oils, and unneeded calories—and the more likely it is that you should step away from the package so no one gets hurt!

There's also strong evidence that, as a rule, the closer to nature you eat, the fewer calories it will take for you to feel satisfied. The reason? Processed foods often have low amounts of fiber and water; a high ratio of calories to nutrients; and a mix of tastes from added sugar, salt, and flavoring that overly stimulates the appetite center in the hypothalamus.

Clean foods are the opposite: lots of fiber and fluids, a high ratio of nutrients to calories, and no added flavors—all of which send signals of satiety to your brain before you consume too many calories. For example, think of how many raw almonds you eat before stopping; compare that to honey roasted almonds—that sugary coating spurs you to eat more. By eating clean, you can control your weight permanently without feeling deprived or hungry or having constant cravings.

(continued on page 224)

50 HEALTHIEST EVERYDAY FOODS

The journey from fresh to processed is not a simple one, and eating completely clean at every meal isn't always realistic. That's why we compiled this chart to show how common foods morph from real to highly processed. Your goal: Choose from foods in their natural state as often as possible, go with foods that are somewhat processed in a pinch, and limit highly processed items. Turn to page 228 for smarter packaged choices that make clean cooking easier and more convenient.

NATURAL STATE (FIRST CHOICE)	SOMEWHAT PROCESSED (SECOND CHOICE)	HIGHLY PROCESSED (LIMIT)	SHOPPING TIP
Apple	Applesauce	Apple toaster pastry	Applesauce is a healthy choice, but it has fewer nutrients than a whole apple.
Orange	100% orange juice	Orange drink	Many fruit drinks contain high fructose corn syrup and little real juice.
Strawberries	Strawberry preserves	Strawberry gelatin dessert	Gelatin desserts usually contain artificial strawberry flavor, not real fruit.
Peach	Canned peaches in 100% juice	Canned peaches in heavy syrup	Fruit canned in heavy syrup has more sugar and calories than fresh.
Fresh figs	Fig preserves	Fig sandwich cookies	Packaged fruit cookies may contain refined sugar and preservatives.
Pineapple	Canned diced pineapple	Pineapple cocktail cup	Fresh pineapple is higher in vitamins C and A and beta-carotene than canned.
Corn on the cob	Corn tortilla chips	Cornflakes	Buy tortilla chips with just three ingredients: whole corn, oil, and salt—and eat them in moderation.
Spinach	Bagged prewashed spinach	Frozen creamed spinach	Avoid frozen vegetables in sodium-rich sauces. Buy plain and add your own light sauce.
Garlic	Jarred minced garlic	Bottled garlic marinade	Minced fresh garlic is cheaper and more flavorful than jarred.

NATURAL STATE (FIRST CHOICE)	SOMEWHAT PROCESSED (SECOND CHOICE)	HIGHLY PROCESSED (LIMIT)	SHOPPING TIP
Carrots	Baby carrots	Frozen honey glazed carrots	Baby carrots are healthy but more expensive than regular-size loose carrots.
Soup from scratch	Canned soup	Dehydrated soup mix	Homemade soup often has less sodium and more flavor than canned.
Heritage ham	Deli ham	Packaged deli bologna	Heritage varieties of pork are much less likely to contain hormones than factory meat is.
Whole turkey	Deli turkey	Turkey meatballs	If you buy deli meat, ask for brands free of fillers and nitrates.
Grass-fed beef	Grain-fed beef	Frozen beef patties	Grass-fed meat is higher in nutrients and lower in fat than grain-fed beef.
Fresh chicken breasts	Deli sliced chicken	Chicken nuggets	Chicken nuggets contain very little real chicken.
Pasture-raised eggs	Omega-3 fortified eggs	Egg Beaters	Pasture-raised eggs may have 35% less saturated fat, 60% more vitamin A, and 200% more omega-3s.
Cream	Fat-free half cream/ half milk	Flavored dairy creamers	Flavored dairy creamers are often made with colorings, artificial flavors, and corn syrup.
Plain yogurt	Flavored yogurt	Flavored yogurt drink	Buy plain yogurt and flavor it at home with honey or fresh fruit.
Whole grain bread	Wheat bread	Fortified white bread	If a whole grain isn't the first ingredient, you're missing out on nutrients.
Dried whole wheat pasta	Dried white pasta	Instant noodles	Whole grain pasta is higher in antioxidants than white or instant noodles.
Brown rice	White rice	Flavored instant rice	Brown rice, unlike white, hasn't had its fiber-rich layers of bran and germ removed.
Peanuts	Natural peanut butter	Processed peanut butter	Natural peanut butter should contain only peanuts and a dash of salt.
Fresh edamame	Tofu	Frozen veggie burgers	Frozen veggie burgers are vegetarian friendly but are highly processed.

So, let's sum up the importance of eating clean. Our bodies replace billions of cells every day, using the foods we consume as the source of building materials. Eating well is part of the formula that can reduce our risk of any major chronic disease by 80 percent and have a deep effect of improving the health of our very genes.

Perhaps your parents admonished you, as a child, to clean your plate because there were starving kids in China. These days, China, like us, has epidemic obesity. Forget about cleaning your plate; focus instead on choosing clean foods to put on it in the first place. You know what's at stake: life itself, the liberty that comes with good health, and the likelihood of happiness.

Now that you realize the urgency of clean eating, there's no time to waste! The following nine steps will get you started. Then review page 222 and follow our chart to distinguish whole food from processed food.

NINE EASY WAYS TO CLEAN UP YOUR DIET

Our rules will have you eating less junk and fewer hidden calories, so you can slim down and stay healthy naturally.

Food used to be simple. You ate what you grew on the land or bought from nearby farmers. Processed food was nothing more than canned, frozen, or cured. Today, food is much more complicated, and we're both better and worse off for it. We can eat a greater variety of healthy foods than our ancestors did (think fresh berries in winter), but we also can eat a lot more highly processed, chemical-laden ones. And that fare seems to be winning the day, if our epidemics of obesity and diabetes are any indication.

But an increasing trend toward clean eating—with its emphasis on whole, fresh, traditional fare—could mark a turning point in our sometimes dysfunctional relationship with food and help us achieve good health, culinary satisfaction, and optimal fitness.

To help you clean up your own diet and reap the benefits (weight loss and possible decreased risk of diabetes, heart disease, and cancer), we created these nine rules. You'll be eating clean in no time.

Toss a few heavily processed staples. Instead of overhauling your pantry all at once, start by eliminating corn oil and soda—both highly processed, says Nina Planck, author of *Real Food: What to Eat and Why*. "That alone," she says, "is a huge first step." (Another easy step is replacing refined breads and pastas made from white flour with ones made from whole grains.)

Clean up the biggest part of your diet. To keep it simple, assess what part of your diet supplies the most calories, suggests Mary Ellen Camire, PhD, a professor of food science and nutrition at the University of Maine. If you're an omnivore, buy meat that comes from grass-fed cattle and eggs from pasture-raised chickens, but stick to conventional produce instead of organic. If you're a vegetarian, buying organic produce makes more sense.

Shop the perimeter of the supermarket. Most whole, natural foods are on the outside aisles of grocery stores—that's where the produce, dairy, and meat sections usually are. As you go deeper into the center of the store, you encounter more processed and packaged food. "Find the stuff that spoils," suggests nutritionist Jonny Bowden, PhD, author of *The Most Effective Ways to Live Longer*.

Read labels. It's the easiest way to distinguish a "clean" food from a highly processed one. Think about it: A head of lettuce has no label (totally natural), while a bag of ranch-flavored corn chips has a dozen or more ingredients (highly processed). Instead of eliminating all processed foods, study the labels on the packaging and choose those with fewer and simpler ingredients (avoid hydrogenated oils, artificial flavors and colors, stabilizers, preservatives, excessive amounts of fat and sodium, and added refined sugar).

Think in nutrients per serving. Consider the amount of nutrients in a product rather than focusing solely on price. Ask yourself if the price of the food is worth the nutrients (or lack thereof). You can make this assessment on every item by comparing the protein, fiber, minerals, and vitamins against fat, sodium, sugars, and chemical additives. Some clean eaters also focus on the environmental impact of the food. Some stores are promising to make the assessment easier. Walmart is phasing in a sustainable product index designed to help consumers judge at a glance the environmental impact of products (including food).

A new organization called the Ecological Food Manufacturers Association is pushing companies to go even further. "A consumer should be able to pick up a product and, by looking at one little score, instantly know how safe, planet friendly, and nutritious it is," says EFMA founder and CEO Winston Riley. NuVal (a food rating system designed by Dr. Katz and other medical experts, which gives points to foods based on their nutritional content) is available in more than 500 supermarkets nationwide. The higher the score, the cleaner the food. You can also use your iPhone to access GoodGuide, a free application that offers health, environment, and social responsibility information, plus ratings, on over 50,000 products (or go to www.goodguide.com).

Cook more meals at home. This is an easy way to shift more of your resources toward whole food and potentially save money. Plus, many restaurants rely on highly processed food to create their meals. To make home cooking easier, master a few one-pot or one-pan dishes with simple ingredients that you can whip up quickly and that will feed the family for days.

"In my fridge right now, I have some beef chili and meat loaf," says Planck, a mother of three. "Each makes a wholesome meal with plenty of leftovers." Cooking helps you appreciate and enjoy your food more, especially if you share the process with others, says Michael Pollan, author of *The Omnivore's Dilemma* and *In Defense of Food*. He recommends involving family by giving them a job (wash, chop, stir, set the table, etc.). As a bonus, he notes that people who cook tend to eat more healthfully and weigh less than those who don't.

"When I switched from vegetarian and low-fat to good-quality animal proteins, pasture-raised eggs, fruits, vegetables, and whole grains, I lost weight without feeling hungry or moody," Planck adds.

Adjust your tastebuds. If you're accustomed to eating food with lots of salt, sugar, fat, and other additives, you'll need to retrain your tastebuds to appreciate the more subtle flavors of whole foods. For instance, if you don't immediately like the taste of brown rice, mix it with white (in decreasing amounts) until you adapt. (You can do the same thing with whole grain pasta.)

It works for salty and fatty foods, too. Instead of switching immediately to, say, low-sodium soups, mix a regular can with a low-sodium version and adjust the ratio toward less sodium as you get used to the flavor. It can take up to 12 weeks to adjust, says Richard Mattes, PhD, MPH, a professor of foods and nutrition at Purdue University.

Follow an 80-20 strategy. Eating plans go bad (and are eventually abandoned) when they turn obsessive. Clean eating is no different. To avoid that trap, take an 80-20 approach. That is, try to eat natural food 80 percent of the time, with a 20 percent buffer for when you're traveling or socializing or simply can't.

Feel the love. For Dr. Camire, clean eating is all about the pleasures of food. She remembers some advice that celebrity chef Alton Brown of the Food Network delivered at an Institute of Food Technologists conference a few years ago. "I'll never forget it," she says. "He said, 'You know, as long as it's made with love . . .' That really stuck with me because it goes back to the whole French paradox thing: While the French are talking with family, drinking wine, and turning eating into a celebration, we're scarfing down handheld food in our cars. His message was to think about where your food is coming from, who's preparing it, and especially how you're eating it."

In other words, be mindful. It's a word that comes up repeatedly in discussions of clean eating. Be more mindful of how you shop, how you cook, and how you eat.

"I choose to eat this way for many reasons, and one of the biggest is enjoyment," says Pollan. "There doesn't have to be a trade-off between pleasure and health. If you eat this way, you can have both. This diet is amplifying the voice of your mother, the voices of your grandmothers, and the voice in you. It's not rocket science. In fact, it's not even science. It's just common sense."

PACKAGED FOODS WE LOVE

You don't have to sacrifice convenience or your budget to eat clean. More companies are producing foods that are relatively unprocessed and more healthful. We asked our experts to recommend their favorites—the foods they grab off supermarket shelves when they don't have time to cook from scratch.

Fruits/Veggies

Produce picked and frozen at peak ripeness has just as many nutrients and antioxidants as fresh, if not more.

Dole Wildly Nutritious Signature Blends Frozen Mixed Fruit

Cascadian Farm Organic Frozen Cut Spinach

Cereals

Simplicity is key for these three brands: minimal processing and few additives.

Bear Naked 100% Pure & Natural Cranberry Raisin Cereal

Arrowhead Mills Organic Steel Cut Oats Hot Cereal

Post Shredded Wheat Cereal

Dairy

These brands are made from milk that's free of antibiotics and hormones.

Stonyfield Farm Organic Yogurt

Organic Valley Lowfat 1% Milk

Meals

These items let their ingredients' natural flavors speak for themselves—no refined sugar or excessive fat or salt.

Birds Eye Asparagus Stir-Fry

Annie's Homegrown Organic Whole Wheat Shells and White Cheddar

Kashi All-Natural Tuscan Veggie Bake

Pantry Staples

These products make it easy and delicious to incorporate whole grains and omega-3s into your diet.

Uncle Ben's Fast & Natural Whole Grain Instant Brown Rice

Ronzoni Healthy Harvest Whole Wheat Blend Spaghetti

Colavita Extra Virgin Olive Oil

Pacific Natural Foods Organic Free-Range Chicken Broth

Bumble Bee Skinless and Boneless Pink Salmon

Breads

Sprouted grain bread contains more than twice the dietary fiber of white or wheat bread.

Food for Life Organic 7 Sprouted Grains Bread

Alvarado St. Bakery Sprouted Multi-Grain Bread

Snacks/Condiments/Spreads

From the one ingredient in Crazy Richard's Peanut Butter (peanuts) to the blend of raw fruits, nuts, and spices in the Lärabar, these snacks are as real as processed gets.

Lärabar energy bars

Snyder's of Hanover Sourdough Hard Pretzels

St. Dalfour Black Cherry 100% Fruit Spread

Crazy Richard's Natural Chunky Peanut Butter

Guiltless Gourmet Mild Black Bean Dip

Wholly Guacamole Classic

Sabra Classic Hummus

San Marcos Chipotle Peppers in Adobo Sauce

Drew's All Natural Organic Salsa

Desserts

Häagen-Dazs Fat Free Mango Sorbet

CHAPTER 20

The Best Foods You Can Buy

We gathered some of the biggest names in food and nutrition for our annual roundup of the healthiest, tastiest, and most affordable products on the market

Eating whole, unprocessed food is smart health advice that we're squarely behind, but cooking from scratch every single day can be unrealistic. Imagine a weeknight meal without at least one packaged item (think frozen veggies and a box of pasta).

To strike a balance, we asked five leading nutrition experts for their favorite healthy packaged foods—that means no trans fats, refined grains, high sodium levels, or hidden sugar (or unpronounceable ingredients) and plenty of antioxidants, minerals, whole grains, and good-for-you monounsaturated fats. Our experts gave the thumbs-up to nearly 100 products and the boot to more than 300. In a 4-hour taste test, *Prevention* staffers narrowed it down to 25 favorites (including some great budget buys).

FROZEN VEGETABLES

Alexia Select Sides Roasted Red Potatoes & Baby Portabella Mushrooms

Toss these vitamin-packed spuds, 'shrooms, and green beans into a skillet, stir in the packet of thyme-infused canola and olive oil blend, and cook for 10 minutes.

"I love these nicely seasoned veggies," raves judge Brian Wansink, PhD.

Per 1¼ cups: 140 calories, 7 grams fat, 180 milligrams sodium

FROZEN DINNER WINNERS

TV dinners don't have to be bland to be healthy: A *Consumer Reports* study tested 22 lower-calorie entrées and rated many as "very good" in both taste and nutrition. The only caveat? Most were too low in calories. Eat an extra serving of fruit or veggies to turn these high-ranking choices into satisfying meals.

Best Beef

Healthy Choice Café Steamers Roasted Beef Merlot

WHY IT'S TOPS: Generous chunks of succulent steak in a classic meat-and-potatoes meal that has just 2 grams of saturated fat.

Best Chicken

Kashi Chicken Florentine

WHY IT'S TOPS: White wine and Parmesan cheese toppings add buttery flavor to fiber-rich whole grains.

Best Vegetarian

Lean Cuisine One Dish Favorites Santa Fe–Style Rice & Beans

WHY IT'S TOPS: A mild chile sauce kicks up the flavor of this meatless entrée that provides nearly one-quarter of the protein you need daily. Yee-haw!

FRUIT

Dole Sliced Strawberries

When berries aren't in season, it's great to have a frozen option handy, says judge Cheryl Forberg, RD, who likes this unsweetened brand.

As an added bonus, Dole's berries are frozen shortly after they are picked so they don't lose vitamin C (1 cup has 90 percent of what you need for the day). And even better news: They're loaded with anthocyanins, antioxidants that might help lower cholesterol and reduce your risk of cancer to boot.

Per cup: 50 calories, 0 gram fat, 0 milligram sodium

SWEET POTATO

Mann's Sweet Potato Spears

Do you hate peeling potatoes? We hate it, too. Go for this bag of ready-to-cook fry-shaped sweet tubers. Season with 2 tablespoons olive oil and a little sea salt, and bake for 25 minutes. Simple and delicious!

"These fries feel like a total splurge, but they're nutrient packed," says Forberg. "One serving provides the cancer-fighting vitamin A you need for the day."

Per cup (uncooked): 70 calories, 0 gram fat, 45 milligrams sodium

JUICE

Tropicana Trop50 Pomegranate Blueberry

This fruit juice/water blend is sweetened with stevia, which is a compound that comes from a shrub native to South America, for half the calories of a typical glass.

"Stevia is natural and seems to be free of problems associated with artificial sweeteners," says judge David Katz, MD, MPH.

Per cup: 50 calories, 0 gram fat, 10 milligrams sodium

NOODLES

Bionaturae 100% Organic Whole Wheat Lasagne

Made from whole durum wheat grown on family farms in Italy, these noodles have 6 grams of fiber and 7 grams of protein per serving.

"Plus, the texture and flavor are wonderful," gushes Forberg.

Per 3 noodles: 180 calories, 1.5 grams fat, 0 milligram sodium

OATMEAL

Country Choice Organic Quick Cook Steel Cut Oats

If you prefer the texture (and health benefits) of steel-cut oats to instant oats but don't have time to make them every morning, you'll love this product. This company cracks the whole oat before it's chopped so it cooks in just 5 to 7 minutes. Everything is the same nutritionally—the filling fiber, whole grain, and heart-healthy antioxidants. And does the taste pass muster? Forberg, a longtime steel-cut oatmeal fan, gives it "a big thumbs-up."

Per cup (prepared with water): 150 calories, 3 grams fat, 0 milligram sodium

FROZEN ENTRÉE

Healthy Choice All Natural Roasted Red Pepper Marinara

Budget buy: Our experts thought this affordable entrée was better nutritionally than many of the pricier organic brands. Tasty whole grain pasta is tossed with roasted red pepper sauce and topped with grated cheese. The result: 5 grams of fiber and 15 percent of your daily calcium need, plus at least 10 percent of nine other vitamins and minerals per serving.

"It's a little low in calories and high in sodium," says judge Elisa Zied, RD. "So pair it with a medium apple or banana for another 100 or so calories to keep you satisfied and extra potassium to help balance the sodium in the dish."

Per meal: 270 calories, 6 grams fat, 580 milligrams sodium

RICE

Uncle Ben's Whole Grain White Rice

If you don't like the chewy texture of brown rice but know it's good for you (it has 3 grams of fiber per cup and trace minerals like zinc and copper), you'll flip for this lighter whole grain variety.

"The stealth approach is wonderful," says Dr. Wansink. "It looks like white but has the nutrition of brown."

Per cup (cooked): 170 calories, 1 gram fat, 5 milligrams sodium

CHINESE

Annie Chun's Mini Wontons

For a quick, fun meal, boil these wontons—either the Pork & Ginger or the Chicken & Cilantro—in low-sodium broth.

"Most wonton soups have more than 900 milligrams of sodium," says Zied. "With these, you could make your own for under 300 milligrams." In addition, the company uses antibiotic-free chicken.

Per 4 pieces (Chicken & Cilantro): 50 calories, 0.5 gram fat, 160 milligrams sodium

YOGURT

Chobani Greek Yogurt

All Greek yogurts are thicker, creamier, and have more filling protein in 6 ounces than their American counterparts. But Chobani's fat-free flavors—including the new raspberry—taste "particularly luscious," says Forberg. "It's like eating dessert. Even the plain is amazing."

Another bonus: The company's packaging is widely recyclable, 10 percent of its profits go to charity, and it buys hormone-free milk from a local dairy.

Per 6-ounce carton (raspberry): 140 calories, 0 gram fat, 65 milligrams sodium

EGGS

Eggland's Best Eggs

Already lower in cholesterol and fat than other brands, Eggland's Best eggs now have four times more vitamin D (which helps your body absorb calcium) and three times more omega-3 fatty acids (which lower the risk of sudden heart attacks and may improve your memory). That's because the company removed animal products and added vitamins and minerals to the chicken feed.

"It's smart to use these eggs to help prevent heart trouble," says Dr. Katz. You can buy them in assorted sizes and organically raised.

Per large egg: 70 calories, 4 grams fat, 60 milligrams sodium

SOUP

Campbell's Select Harvest Light Savory Chicken with Vegetables Soup

The broth is packed with veggies, which supply a bounty of antioxidants and 60 percent of the vitamin A you need daily.

"The colorful veggies make this more special than typical canned soup," says Zied. Chicken breast pieces pump up the protein (5 grams per serving), while sea salt adds more flavor than regular salt, so the company didn't use as much.

Per cup: 80 calories, 1 gram fat, 480 milligrams sodium

CRACKERS

Triscuit Thin Crisps

Budget buy: Made only with fiber-rich whole wheat, soybean and/or palm oil, and salt, these triangle-shaped crackers are more airy than regular Triscuits and many of the more expensive health food store brands.

"You get about twice as many crackers for the same number of calories," says Zied.

Per 15 pieces: 130 calories, 5 grams fat, 180 milligrams sodium

MEET OUR GRADE-A EXPERTS

SUGAR SLEUTH: Nutritionist for NBC's *The Biggest Loser* and coauthor of *The Biggest Loser: 6 Weeks to a Healthier You,* Cheryl Forberg, RD, vetoed more foods than any judge.

NUTRIENT GURU: Director of the Yale Prevention Research Center and codeveloper of the NuVal Nutritional Scoring System, David L. Katz, MD, MPH, ensured the picks weren't empty calories.

TASTER-IN-CHIEF: Author of the much-beloved *Moosewood Cookbook,* Mollie Katzen gave us her gourmet opinion. Her latest book, *Get Cooking,* is especially for culinary novices.

REALITY CHECKER: Director of Cornell University Food and Brand Lab and author of *Mindless Eating,* Brian Wansink, PhD, is a regular at McDonald's and Sam's Club. He kept us all grounded.

CALORIE COUNTER: Foods with sneaky hidden calories had no chance with Elisa Zied, RD, spokesperson for the American Dietetic Association and author of *Nutrition at Your Fingertips.*

DELI MEAT

Hormel Natural Choice Mesquite Deli Turkey

Budget buy: This brand has about one-third less sodium than many others on the shelf.

"If you eat deli meat a few times a week, it's especially important to choose a low-sodium version," says Zied. Another plus: It leaves out the nitrates or preservatives (some research has linked nitrates to colon cancer) without charging you a premium.

Per 3-slice serving: 50 calories, 1 gram fat, 450 milligrams sodium

TOFU

Nasoya Organic TofuPlus

Budget buy: All tofu contains heart-healthy isoflavones, but this brand is fortified with B vitamins and vitamin D, plus 20 percent of your daily calcium need—and doesn't cost more than regular tofu.

"Women's calcium requirements go up by 200 milligrams when they hit 51, so switching to this tofu can help make up the difference," says Zied. "Extra vitamin B_{12} is also helpful because you don't absorb as much after age 50."

Per 3-ounce serving: 70 calories, 3 grams fat, 0 milligram sodium

BURGER

SeaPak Salmon Burgers

These patties are rich in omega-3s, fats that protect the heart and may help battle depression and—early research suggests—might help you lose weight.

"These are great for people who don't like the strong flavor or texture of a salmon fillet," says Dr. Katz, who enjoyed the smoky taste and meat loaf consistency. And the salmon is wild and sustainably caught.

Per burger: 110 calories, 3 grams fat, 380 milligrams sodium

APPLESAUCE

Santa Cruz Organic Apple Peach Sauce

Adding peaches to applesauce delivers vitamins A and E and different kinds of anthocyanins, cancer-fighting antioxidants.

"It's an easy way to add more variety to your diet because nutrients work in synergy," says Zied. You can find it in jars or preportioned cups.

Per ½ cup: 80 calories, 0 gram fat, 10 milligrams sodium

CHEESE

Laughing Cow Mini Babybel Light

Packed with 200 milligrams of calcium apiece, these mini rounds are made with part-skim milk, which saves 2.5 grams of artery-clogging saturated fat. Dr. Wansink likes that they're double wrapped.

"It takes a minute to open, so you're not eating it mindlessly and you may eat less," he says.

Per piece: 50 calories, 3 grams fat, 160 milligrams sodium

FROZEN YOGURT

Blue Bunny Double Raspberry All Natural Frozen Yogurt

Budget buy: This yogurt tastes like raspberry soft-serve ice cream with about 20 fewer calories, one-third the fat, and more calcium.

"Be sure to stick to a half-cup portion," reminds Zied. "A half gallon of this is roughly the same price as a pint of premium ice cream, but with the bigger package, it's easy to get carried away."

Per ½ cup: 110 calories, 2 grams fat, 50 milligrams sodium

SORBET

Häagen-Dazs Mango All Natural Sorbet Cups

Single-serve containers are the solution to "just one more bite" syndrome. The satisfying portion (a tad more than ½ cup) comes with a little spoon tucked under the lid.

"It has a good, real mango flavor," says judge Mollie Katzen. Thanks to that mango, one serving supplies 15 percent of the vitamin A and 10 percent of the vitamin C you need daily.

Per container: 140 calories, 0 gram fat, 0 milligram sodium

CHOCOLATE TOPPING

Justin's All-Natural Chocolate Hazelnut Butter

This spread made from organic cocoa (which has more heart-healthy flavonoids than tea or wine) and dry-roasted hazelnuts (packed with vitamin E and high in good-for-you monounsaturated fats) will totally satisfy.

"It has a slightly salty nut flavor with just a hint of sweetness from the chocolate," says Katzen, who tried it as a dip with fruit and on a sliver of sourdough bread. It also comes in preportioned 80-calorie packets.

Per 2 tablespoons: 190 calories, 16 grams fat, 75 milligrams sodium

PESTO SAUCE

Le Grand Garden Pesto Sauce

Made with two herbs—basil (its oils might contain anti-inflammatory compounds) and parsley (packed with vitamin K for strong bones)—this sauce has plenty of monounsaturated fats from canola oil. It also has a better herb-to-oil ratio than most other pestos, sparing you about 40 calories for every 2 tablespoons.

"It tastes like it was made from the herbs in your backyard," says Katzen, who fell head over heels for it.

Per 2 tablespoons: 110 calories, 12 grams fat, 210 milligrams sodium

TOMATO-BASIL SAUCE

Monte Bene Farm Fresh Tomato Basil Pasta Sauce

Budget buy: A lower-priced version of the company's gourmet brand, this sauce relies on tasty, locally grown tomatoes for sweetness rather than sugar or, even worse, high fructose corn syrup.

"It's hard to find a mainstream brand that hasn't been sweetened," says Zied, who made delicious spaghetti and meatballs with this sauce. Another thing Zied liked: It has about one-half to one-third of the sodium in other brands.

Per ½ cup: 24 calories, 1 gram fat, 191 milligrams sodium

SEASONING

Mrs. Dash Fiesta Lime Seasoning Blend

Budget buy: A dozen spices such as cumin, coriander, oregano, and rosemary go into this mix.

"Spices contain different antioxidants—some benefit the heart, some are cancer fighting, others are linked to preventing diabetes—so a blend is a super way to get the variety," says Zied. Salt free, this blend is a lot less expensive (and healthier) than gourmet.

Per ¼ teaspoon: 0 calorie, 0 gram fat, 0 milligram sodium

GRILL SAUCE

Spectrum Organic Malay Asam Grill and Finishing Sauce

Try this citrusy marinade (a blend of pineapple juice, soy oil, soy sauce, and anti-inflammatory spices like turmeric and ginger) to add zing to grilled meat or fish or a chicken stir-fry.

"It's also a great alternative to high-sodium soy sauce for dipping," says Dr. Katz.

Per 2 tablespoons: 50 calories, 4 grams fat, 160 milligrams sodium

CHAPTER 21

Hidden Expiration Dates

Are your nutrients expiring? Here's how to store olive oil, potatoes, and other staples so they retain their extraordinary healing powers

Common products in your kitchen have an expiration date that doesn't appear on the package—the day their nutrients start downgrading. Here's how to store foods so that you don't miss out on their beneficial nutrients.

When meat smells funky or fruit gets moldy, you know it's time to toss it. But new science is showing that even "nonperishables" such as tea, olive oil, dried herbs, and grains can lose valuable nutrients during months in your pantry. We surveyed a dozen experts to find out what's at risk, and we learned some tips for prolonging your food's nutritional shelf life.

GREEN TEA

Antioxidants decrease an average of 32 percent after 6 months on the shelf, according to a 2009 study in the *Journal of Food Science*. These antioxidants, known as catechins, might decrease your risk of several types of cancer, but they are sensitive to both oxygen and light. Sadly, tea, unlike wine, does not improve with age.

Make it last: "Buy tea in airtight packages such as tins, rather than cellophane wraps, which air can penetrate," advises Rona Tison of ITO EN, the world's largest supplier of green tea. Store your tea bags in sealed, opaque canisters in a cool spot. "Green tea is more sensitive to heat than black tea, so place your sealed container in the refrigerator to keep the leaves fresh and healthy for as long as possible," she says.

TOMATO PRODUCTS

Canned tomato juice loses 50 percent of its lycopene after 3 months in the refrigerator—even when it's unopened, says a study in *Food Chemistry.* Similarly, scientists in Spain have found that the lycopene in ketchup deteriorates over time. That's a shame, because it's a potent antioxidant that might fight many forms of cancer and heart disease and even strengthen bones.

Make it last: Skip the premade tomato sauce and make your own using boxed whole or diced tomatoes rather than pureed. Whole and diced tomatoes contain more solids, which provide added protection for the lycopene, says B. H. Chen, PhD, a food scientist at Fu Jen University in Taiwan who analyzes the stability of carotenoids. If ketchup sits in your fridge for months, buy smaller bottles, says Christine Gerbstadt, MD, RD. Fresh bottles tend to start off with higher levels of lycopene.

POTATOES

Vitamin C declined 40 percent, on average, after 8 months in proper storage (in a place that's cool, dark, and dry), according to researchers in Holland. You probably wouldn't keep potatoes that long. But farmers often store them up to 5 months before shipping them to market, says Peter

Imle, a potato farmer and plant geneticist in northern Minnesota.

Make it last: Look for smaller potatoes (often labeled "new"), which have a slightly higher vitamin C content to begin with, and buy only what you can eat in a few weeks. Imle also recommends keeping potatoes in paper sacks, rather than plastic grocery bags.

"Paper keeps out excess light and oxygen. But it still allows the potatoes to breathe, without trapping in moisture like plastic can," he explains.

TWO DRINKS THAT LOSE THEIR PUNCH

Similar to foods, beverages can lose their nutrients quickly, too.

Refrigerated Fruit Juices

According to researchers at Arizona State University, the vitamin C in OJ diminishes by almost 50 percent after just 7 days open in the fridge—most likely because the cartons are not airtight (even those with screw-on caps). Separate studies show that the nutrients in canned tomato and mango juices also decline over time.

MAKE IT LAST: Buy frozen orange juice concentrate, which starts with higher levels of C, and drink it in a week.

Milk and Dairy Products

Fat-free milk in transparent glass bottles loses more than 10 percent of its immunity-boosting vitamin A after just 2 hours in the dairy case, according to the *Journal of Dairy Science*. And the riboflavin in cheese depletes drastically when exposed to fluorescent lights, like those in most retail shops, say Danish researchers.

MAKE IT LAST: Buy milk in cartons and cheese wrapped in waxed paper rather than clear plastic. Store cheese in an opaque drawer.

OLIVE OIL

The potency of antioxidants declined 40 percent after 6 months, according to a 2009 Italian study of bottled olive oil in the *Journal of Food Science*. Yet in many households, bottles can sit on the shelf for much longer than that.

Make it last: Don't store oil near the stove or leave it uncapped for long, because it's sensitive to oxygen, heat, and light, says Doug Balentine, PhD, director of nutrition sciences at Unilever, which produces Bertolli olive oil. If you don't cook with it often, buy smaller bottles.

BERRY JAMS

The anthocyanins in blueberry jam decline by 23 percent, on average, after 2 months of storage at room temperature, say researchers at the University of Arkansas. Similarly, strawberry jam loses up to 12 percent of its health-boosting flavonoids after 6 months in a dark cupboard. Experts believe the flavonoids (including anthocyanins) contribute to the anti-inflammatory, memory-preserving, antioxidant effects of berries.

Make it last: Store jams in the fridge before opening to retain about 15 percent more of the anthocyanins and their antiaging benefits. Or buy sugar-free blueberry jams. Researchers found that they maintain higher levels of anthocyanins over time.

DRIED HERBS AND SPICES

The capsaicin in chili powder decreased continuously during 9 months of storage in one Chinese study. Capsaicin might contribute to weight loss and also help fight certain cancers.

"Generally, spices that should be bright in color but have grown dull are also devoid of flavor and nutritional value," says Jay Bunting, owner of Wayzata Bay Spice Co.

Make it last: Buy in glass jars whenever possible, says Bunting. (Air penetrates plastic.) Better yet, grind your own. Whole spices such as peppercorns retain health benefits and flavor much longer because the inside of each peppercorn is protected from light and air. Store herbs and spices out of direct light and away from the hot stove.

GRAINS AND DRY GOODS

The riboflavin in enriched macaroni plummeted 50 percent after being exposed to light for only a day, according to a *Journal of Food Science* study. Even dim light can degrade riboflavin by 80 percent after 3 months, according to another study. The folic acid in enriched flour is also sensitive to both light and oxygen.

Make it last: Store grains in opaque ceramic containers, far from the stove's damaging heat. A dry cupboard is better than the fridge, except in the case of brown rice, which contains a small amount of oil and therefore spoils faster at room temperature.

CHAPTER 22

Is Your Food Making You Old?

Feeling fatigued, forgetful, or achy? Don't automatically chalk it up to getting older. These easy fixes might turn back the clock

What if the fountain of youth were in your own kitchen? While we've come to expect that certain physical and mental changes are an inevitable part of getting older, the fact is that the foods we eat—or don't—might speed those processes along, aging us before our time.

The reason is simple. "We eat too many processed foods," says David Katz, MD, MPH, director of Yale University's Prevention Research Center. "They're often high in calories and low in nutrients such as vitamin B_{12} and omega-3s, so we end up with islands of deficiencies in a sea of excess."

These inadequacies can result in symptoms we tend to assume are due to aging, such as the four in this chapter. Work with your doctor to determine whether adjusting your diet or adding a supplement can help you look—and feel—younger.

YOU HAVE LESS ENERGY

You might need more: Vitamin B_{12}

Found only in foods that are derived from animals, this nutrient helps regulate your metabolism and energy production and is key to maintaining a healthy brain and nervous system.

"Fatigue is a classic sign of B_{12} deficiency, which usually occurs in people who don't eat very much animal protein," says Danine Fruge, MD, associate medical director of the Pritikin Longevity Center & Spa in Miami. Chewing a lot of antacids to relieve heartburn can also lead to B_{12} deficiency, because antacids interfere with B_{12} absorption.

How your doctor knows: Your GP will ask about what you eat, whether you're getting enough sleep, and the medications you take. If you don't eat many (or any) meat or dairy foods or take supplements containing B_{12}, you sleep 7 to 8 hours each night, and you're physically active, odds are good that your low energy is due to a B_{12} deficiency.

Food fix: Have two servings of fat-free dairy foods, such as fat-free milk or fat-free yogurt, and 3 to 4 ounces of lean protein daily. Good sources of B_{12} include seafood such as fish, clams, oysters, and mussels, as well as lean beef and pork, chicken, and fortified cereal.

Supplement solution: Take 500 to 1,000 micrograms of vitamin B_{12} in tablet form every day to raise and maintain your B_{12} levels.

YOUR JOINTS ACHE

You might need more: Manganese and copper

Because manganese and copper are both essential for maintaining joint cartilage and flexibility, "in most cases, supplementing these nutrients reverses the joint deterioration and eliminates the pain," says Dale Peterson, MD, director of the Comprehensive Wellness Center in Sapulpa, Oklahoma. "The body can actually repair a significant amount of damage if it's given the proper support."

How your doctor knows: Using a simple blood test, your physician can easily determine whether your joint pain is related to garden-variety wear and tear or a more serious inflammatory condition.

"If the result is normal, you can be assured that the joint pain isn't caused by serious rheumatic disease," says Dr. Peterson.

Food fix: Nuts, beef, and spinach are good sources of these nutrients, but you won't be able to eat enough to get all your copper and manganese, so opt for a supplement, Dr. Peterson advises.

Supplement solution: Take 2 milligrams of copper and 5 milligrams of manganese each day. Within 2 to 3 months, your joints should feel less painful.

YOU'RE MORE FORGETFUL

You might need more: Omega-3 essential fatty acids

"These fatty acids are part of the brain's building blocks," explains Andrew Weil, MD, director of the Arizona Center for Integrative Medicine at the University of Arizona. "If you're not getting enough in your diet, the architecture of the brain becomes weak, and brain function, including memory, suffers."

But it's not only the amount of omega-3s that's important; the balance between omega-3s and omega-6s is equally crucial. "Our diets are flooded with omega-6 fatty acids, mostly from processed foods," says Dr. Weil. "The more omega-6s you eat, the more omega-3s you need to balance your levels. Most of us aren't eating enough omega-3s and are eating too many omega-6s."

How your doctor knows: A quick review of what you eat is all she needs. "If there's no fish, walnuts, or freshly ground flaxseed in your diet, and the fats you eat come mainly from meat, you're not getting any omega-3s," explains Manuel Villacorta, RD, an American Dietetic Association spokesperson in San Francisco.

Food fix: First, reduce the amount of refined and processed foods you eat as much as possible, and cook with olive or canola oil. Then, eat $3\frac{1}{2}$ ounces of wild salmon and $3\frac{1}{2}$ ounces of herring, sardines, or halibut each week. Add

2 tablespoons of freshly ground flaxseed to cereal, whole grain side dishes, or shakes daily, and garnish salads or cereal with 1 tablespoon of walnuts 5 days a week. Finally, enjoy 9 to 12 almonds four times a week.

Supplement solution: Take at least 2,000 milligrams of fish oil daily. Look for 1,000-milligram capsules of combined docosahexaenoic acid (DHA) and eicosaentaenoic acid (EPA).

YOUR BLOOD PRESSURE IS RISING

You might need more: Potassium

"Having too little potassium in your diet magnifies the toxic effects of excessive salt intake," Dr. Fruge says. Most processed foods have added sodium but no extra potassium, so if your meals come from boxes, you're likely at risk. Worsening the situation, when your kidneys try to flush out the salt, you lose even more potassium. "The imbalance damages blood vessels, driving up blood pressure," Dr. Fruge notes. "Eating better can correct the problem. I've seen people drop 30 points in 3 days."

How your doctor knows: A review of your diet reveals all your GP needs to know. If there's any doubt, he can evaluate your cardiovascular function with blood tests to check blood sugar, cholesterol levels, and kidney function, along with stress tests, body-fat measurements, and ultrasounds of your heart and arteries.

Food fix: Cut your sodium consumption to no more than 1,500 milligrams per day, and eat seven to nine servings of fruits and vegetables every day.

Supplement solution: Potassium supplements can lead to arrhythmia or other cardiac problems, says Dr. Fruge. Stick with produce to avoid those side effects.

journal

"I GOT HEALTHY FOR MY FAMILY"

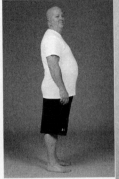

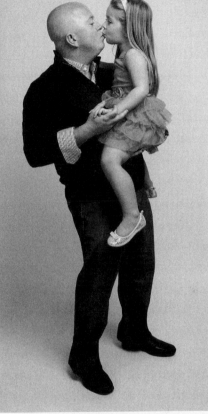

As my weight climbed, so did my wife's concern for my health. Here's the eating plan that helped me shed two sizes in 1 month

by Anthony Henry

When I met my future wife in 2003, I had just graduated from the New York City Fire Department Academy and was in the best shape of my life. But starting work changed that. The heart of the firehouse is in the kitchen, and we often ate rich, elaborate meals.

Two years later, my wife, Beth, was pregnant with our first daughter, and my weight had risen by 40 pounds. With a child on the way, my wife was worried about my health and our family's future. By 2007, I had gained nearly 70 pounds—and the fad diets I kept trying didn't make a difference.

My wake-up call came when I had a doctor's checkup for a new life insurance policy. Not only was I considered obese, but my cholesterol was high, and my blood sugar numbers put me in prediabetes territory. A month after the exam, my wife discovered she was pregnant again. Her fears became unbearable. She was just as worried about me having a heart attack on the job as being injured in a fire.

Fortunately, her fears were allayed when I heard about a new diet for men that *Prevention* was testing, modeled after the successful Flat Belly Diet. The main tenets of the plan: Eat often, control your portions and caloric intake, and include foods rich in monounsaturated fatty acids (MUFAs, for short) in every meal—which studies show help you store less fat in your belly.

Right away, I knew this program was different. You don't have to give up the things you love; you just have to eat healthier portions.

I took a little ribbing at the firehouse at first. But when they saw how hard I was working, they stopped busting my chops and started helping. Before food shopping, they ask what I can eat and how they can make it healthier. The plates are still he-man size, but I'm managing portions, eating about half of what I used to.

By the end of the month-long program, I had lost 27 pounds and 3 inches from my waist. But the biggest change is my outlook. The extra pounds felt insurmountable, but I don't feel helpless anymore. And my entire family is benefiting from my newfound focus on health. We're more active, taking the kids to different parks to play. Nowadays, I walk and jog to pick up Ella from the babysitter a mile away, taking the stroller instead of the car, and I'm even riding my bike again.

Having regained my firefighting physique, I'm setting big goals—like running a half-marathon and raising $50,000 for the Crohn's and Colitis Foundation along the way. My other plan? Get myself in good enough shape to strike a pose in the New York City Firefighter Hunks calendar.

Pinup boy or not, my progress couldn't have made my wife happier: "This was a huge turning point, and I do think it's saved his life."

Here are my top tips:

COOK MORE. The tough part for me was learning to plan my own meals. To get me started, my wife packed food I could take to work. After picking up a few tips from her, I took over. I cooked extras of my favorites, like black and red bean chili, so I'd have leftovers.

PLAN AHEAD. I also learned to make simple staples, such as grilled chicken breasts, to use throughout the week.

ENJOY MUFAS. Beth started putting avocados (a belly-flattening MUFA) on just about everything. Even picky 3-year-old Ella dabbled in MUFAs, sampling almonds and cashews with her breakfast.

Part5

MIND
MATTERS

CHAPTER 23

The Long View of a Healthy Life

Medical journalist Michael Segell draws on decades of experience and perspective to reveal what happy, healthy people have in common

As a health journalist, I've found few analytical tools to be handier than what I call the long view. When whipsawed by "groundbreaking" research that contradicts studies from, oh, just a few weeks before, I find that if I mix the new information into the old, then sit back and wait patiently while it ferments and settles, eventually something I might call truth will rise above the mists of the churning scientific cauldron.

The long view reveals other verities as well. I've always been fascinated by people who enjoy truly outstanding physical and mental health. After years of snooping, I've identified certain behaviors and attitudes they all share—a lifestyle, or style of living, that transcends the healthy habits (Eat this, bend that!) we extol in *Prevention* each month. Here's what my notes—and the long view—tell me about the world's most robust inhabitants.

THEY POSSESS BODY WISDOM

On a reporting trip years ago in California, I interviewed a group of body workers—experts in physical therapies such as the Alexander Technique, Rolfing, and shiatsu—at the Esalen Institute, that epicenter of self-actualization in Big Sur. One therapist, Richard, boasted that he knew of an "inner body" trick that rendered him as implacable as a tree. To demonstrate, he stood before me, assumed a casual stance, then imagined (he told me later) that he had roots that extended deep into Earth's molten core. He told me to shove him—again, harder, and again. Finally, I took a couple of steps back and slammed my shoulder into his. Nothing. Though I outweighed him by 30 pounds, I couldn't budge him. He was a redwood. (And I was in pain!)

Richard had what I call body wisdom. Although his "trick" was probably as much mental as physical, he had a deep awareness of how his body worked and what it was capable of. I've since met many other people I consider bodywise, and while they're not gifted in the physical-stunt category, they are capable of an equally impressive feat: maintaining truly extraordinary health.

YOU'RE MOST LIKELY TO BE HAPPY IF . . .

YOU HAVE A SISTER. People who had at least one female sibling reported better social support, more optimism, and greater coping abilities, according to a study by the British Psychological Society. Sisters appear to encourage cohesion in families.

YOU WERE A SMILEY STUDENT. Adults who had the biggest grins in their college yearbook pictures were up to five times less likely to be divorced decades later than those who looked less happy, according to a new DePauw University study. A smiler's positivity may rub off on a spouse.

YOU'RE NOT GLUED TO THE TV. The happiest people spend 30 percent less time watching the tube, preferring to socialize, read, or attend religious services—habits that are linked to better moods and health.

BE VACATION HAPPY ALL YEAR LONG

S imply thinking about your next getaway may put an extra spring in your step. Dutch researchers found that people who had upcoming vacations scheduled were happier than those without a trip booked, but happiness levels of the two groups were about equal after the travelers returned. It could be that the anticipation of upcoming travel accounts for the mood lift, meaning that a few short weekend excursions throughout the year could make you just as content as a pricier 2-week junket.

Interestingly, most trace the dawning of their physical self-awareness to a minor injury, such as a sprained ankle. A few say they first turned their focus on themselves during a drawn-out struggle with weight, shyness, or stress. What happens next, though, is fairly predictable: They school themselves in basic precepts of nutrition, exercise, and self-healing and design a diet and fitness plan for themselves. As time goes on, they realize that their plan requires regular rethinking. Their bodies change, and their needs do, too. With each updating of their routine, they pay closer attention to its results—a process that deepens their body wisdom.

Their ultimate payoff is an ability to understand their body's unique language. This fluency enables them to recognize when they are depleted, and they rest. They can quickly identify signs of agitation and calm themselves. Their keen awareness and long experience allow them to visualize how their cells are revitalized by specific foods, how the bunched and inflamed fibers of a calf muscle are elongated and soothed by stretching and kneading, and how their flagging brain cells will respond to strong sunlight or a power walk with a mood-boosting squirt of dopamine.

They become body savants, as implacable in their commitment to conscious living as Richard the redwood.

THEY LOVE PHYSICAL PLEASURE

During my college years, I worked during the summers for a fellow named Sean who owned a moving company. Then in his fifties, Sean loved the heavy work; a short, muscular fireplug of a man, he would often tell me that hard physical labor was one of the great pleasures in life, a belief I've held ever since. As we lugged sofas and pianos up and down stairs, he would dispense a torrent of advice in his lilting Irish brogue: Lift with your legs, never eat unless you're hungry, call your parents often, marry young, have as many kids as your wife can bear. A couple of times I almost caused serious injury to us both, I was laughing so hard.

Not long ago, some 35 years after our last moving trip, I visited Sean during a visit to my college town. He invited me onto his porch and poured us both a couple of fingers of Jameson's. He was largely unchanged—spry, still powerfully built, his eyes clear and sparkling as he cracked wise about New England sports teams, town politics, and the stupidity of Twitter, which his grandkids had told him about. I was about to ask him the secret of his remarkable vitality when his wife of untold decades joined us on the porch. As she stood beside him, he affectionately patted her behind, then winked at me.

"If I didn't give Mother a little goose now and then, she'd think I was ready for the winding sheet," he said. Question answered.

Work and love . . . Freud said if you can be successful in both—even if the work is really hard—you'll be happy. Healthy, too. As Sean would attest, the two are intimately connected.

THEY VIEW GOOD HEALTH AS A MORAL OBLIGATION

One (cynical) view of people who take excellent care of themselves, who strive to live as long and well as possible, is that they are narcissists. Certainly, many benefits redound to someone who pursues an intensely healthful lifestyle— not the least of which is that she'll look really good. But from what I've seen, the superhealthy aren't simply on a competitive mission to outlive their friends or become medical marvels. They consider it wrong, in a moral sense,

YOUR HEALTH RULES

When we asked *Prevention* readers how they stay healthy, the advice poured in. Here are our favorites.

Make time for friends. Mine keep me sane.—Christi Bruce

Eat vegetable soup for lunch. I do most days because it's an easy way to up my veggie servings. A big pot made over the weekend lasts me all week.—Kyle Farneski

Spend as much time outdoors as possible.—Rebecca Garson

Stay married—even better for my husband's health, but it's good for mine, too.—Judith Hill

No excuses! My husband and I ride our stationary exercise bike every day when we're home (at least 2 to 4 hours a day). We keep it in the living room so we can ride while we watch TV.—Doris Buchmann

Eat only what tastes really good, which means I don't often eat overprocessed foods.—J. H.

As they say, "Everything in moderation, including moderation."—Donna Agajanian

Wake up and thank the Lord that you can walk and talk. This positive mood spreads to others. Even grumpy people want positive energy coming their way!—Jane Krupica

Volunteer (especially with children). The work keeps me physically active and emotionally grounded. Some of the most remarkable people I know I've met through volunteer work.—Danielle Kosecki

Sign up for long races. They keep you motivated to keep working out. It's not much fun to run in a race for which you haven't properly prepared.—K. F.

not to take care of themselves. Life is a gift, they feel—and one that can be rescinded at any time. To live irresponsibly is to dishonor that gift.

So at the heart of their zeal for health is genuine, life-affirming joy. They wring as much pleasure from every day as they can. A wonderful feedback loop results: To do the things they love, they commit to staying well, get stronger in the process, and end up being able to do even more of the things that enhance their deep appreciation of life.

In taking responsibility for their well-being, they're trying to avoid becoming a burden, in their later years, to those they love. But their health quest is munificent in another way, too. Some of the most interesting epidemiological research to emerge in the past couple of years shows that good health habits are infectious. Scientists have learned, for instance, that if you're a nonsmoker, cheerful, and of a normal weight, your neighbors are likely to be, too.

The world's healthiest people lead by example, fostering good habits in others—even though they begin their campaign by focusing on themselves.

THEY TAKE THE HIT AS A GIFT

Several years ago, a good friend, Lisa, then in her early fifties and in seemingly perfect health, learned she had a dreadful cancer. Her prognosis was not good—only about 10 percent of patients diagnosed with her particular tumor make it to the 5-year mark. Facing two rounds of chemotherapy sandwiched between a double mastectomy and reconstruction, she thought hard about how to respond to her new circumstance.

When she was younger, she had briefly studied the martial art aikido and recalled a favorite saying of her teacher: "Take the hit as a gift." That is, when you suffer a blow—whether from an opponent on the mat or a cluster of

MONEY CAN BUY HAPPINESS!

And it may not cost as much as you think. British psychologists found that the happiness gained from a course of psychotherapy (cost: $1,300) was equivalent to that from a pay raise of more than $41,000. When we buy "stuff," we get temporary happiness, but what you learn about yourself during therapy can have benefits that last the rest of your life, says study author Chris Boyce, PhD.

aggressive cancer cells—redirect the energy from the pain you feel to help you handle whatever you're facing.

So Lisa devised an active counterstrategy: Immediately after receiving her chemo infusion, she would attend a yoga class to work the "medicine"—she refused to call it poison—deep into her tissues. Then, over the next few days, she would go for long walks in the park, even when nauseated, and visualize the demise of the rogue cells in her body. She would harvest the disease's negative power, turning her fear into resolve, her anxiety into hope and confidence.

I've seen other supremely healthy people deploy this strategy in far less extreme circumstances. They view the inevitable upsets and hard knocks in life as "teachable moments"—opportunities to reexamine priorities and strike out in new directions. Some experts would call this resilience, but I prefer to think of it as an ability to take the long view. Change is part of life, and by embracing it we can convert its roiling energy into a source of personal empowerment.

Enlightenment, too: I'll never forget what Lisa told me right after her diagnosis. Processing her new uncertain status was "interesting," she said—she realized, for instance, how full her life had been and was grateful for the insight. She'd had "big love," great kids, a rewarding spiritual life, and a gratifying career. "I've hit all the high notes in life," she told me. "For the sake of my family, I don't want to go, but I'll have no regrets, no unfulfilled yearnings, if I do. The disease has shown me that."

She took the hit as a gift—and it keeps on giving. A dozen years later, her life is even fuller than before.

CHAPTER 24

Breakthrough Mind Games That Help Your Health

The brain has the power to heal the body, and it also has the power to harm. New research reveals why, and how to tip the balance back in your favor

It's a well-researched fact that your thoughts strongly influence your well-being. For instance, consider the placebo response: A pill makes you well just because you believe it will—even if the pill (unbeknownst to you) is made only of sugar.

Unfortunately, your brain can wield an equally negative influence. A classic example: You feel achy and sweaty from the flu you "caught" after getting an influenza shot (even though the virus used in the vaccine is dead). Another: You read about tainted produce and immediately get a stomachache.

This so-called "nocebo effect" also trades on the power of suggestion, duping you into thinking you're ill when you're perfectly fine. Here's how the nocebo effect typically exerts its influence—and how you can outsmart it.

YOU READ ABOUT POTENTIAL SIDE EFFECTS

. . . and you develop them.

While you're smart to stay informed, you might induce or intensify side effects by poring over scary language in a medication insert or reading online about strangers' bad experiences. Keep in mind the FDA requires drug manufacturers to report any side effect experienced during a clinical trial, explains pharmacist Norman Tomaka, CRPh, president of the Florida Pharmacy Association. Even if just 1 percent of trial participants reported insomnia or heartburn, those symptoms will be listed on an insert.

"If a patient happens to be particularly anxious, there's a good chance she'll develop side effects based on what she's read," says Richard Kradin, MD, an associate professor of medicine at Harvard Medical School and author of *The Placebo Response and the Power of Unconscious Healing.* "People naturally tend to experience an imagined outcome," he explains—a process mediated by actual changes in brain neurotransmitters such as dopamine, serotonin, and opioids, which affect our sense of well-being.

Outsmart it: Talk with your pharmacist, who can help you assess and understand your true risk of side effects. For example, Tomaka says many patients are concerned that anti-inflammatory steroids will cause stomach upset, based on reports from friends. A pharmacist can examine your dose, additional medications, and medical history and predict the likelihood that you'll experience the same.

YOU FEAR A SLOW RECOVERY AFTER A PROCEDURE

. . . and it becomes a self-fulfilling prophecy.

Pessimistic thoughts can jump-start a bad experience. "If you go in for a root canal expecting the worst, pain can become even more intense," explains

Guy H. Montgomery, PhD, director of the Integrative Behavioral Medicine Program at Mount Sinai School of Medicine. In one study, he found that emotional distress prior to breast cancer surgery contributed to postsurgical nausea and pain. And in the Framingham Heart Study, women who believed they were destined to develop heart disease were almost four times more likely to die of a heart attack than those who didn't—despite having the same risk factors, explains Elaine D. Eaker, ScD, an epidemiologist who led the study.

Outsmart it: Focus on a positive outcome. Diagnosed with a bulging disk? Seek advice from back-pain patients who improved through yoga or physical therapy. Elevate your expectations by identifying a stress-relieving activity that may work for you. Hypnosis, for one, reduces stress before surgery, says Dr. Montgomery, but anything that calms you, such as meditation, can be helpful.

YOU HEAR ABOUT A HEALTH SCARE IN THE NEWS

. . . and think you're next.

If you've ever read a lice-outbreak bulletin from your child's school and then started itching or heard about tainted tomatoes after eating a BLT and felt queasy, you've experienced this kind of communal nocebo effect.

"At any point, we all have symptoms that we typically ignore—simple things like an itch or ache," says Robin DiMatteo, PhD, a professor of psychology at the University of California, Riverside. But when something like a salmonella outbreak is in the news, our awareness of otherwise benign symptoms is heightened. Blame it on group psychology: Thoughts and emotions, like illnesses, are contagious, Dr. DiMatteo says. That's why you may mistakenly attribute your itchy skin to "the rash" that's going around.

Outsmart it: Assess your symptoms rationally. You need to monitor your environment so you don't ignore a real problem (such as sending your child to the home of a friend with lice). Instead of chalking up a stomachache to tainted produce, ask yourself if you felt ill already. During any outbreak, practice good preventive measures, such as washing your hands and avoiding sick friends. Positive moves will protect your immunity and also help banish a fatalistic sensibility.

CHAPTER 25

A New Me!

Three women discovered calm, confidence, and a positive outlook with our experts' 4-week personality makeovers

Many people assume they're stuck with dyed-in-the-wool traits like shyness, pessimism, and fretfulness. But recent studies from Stanford University and other top institutions show that change is possible. "It's a matter of shifting your thinking," says Leslie Sokol, PhD, a cognitive psychologist at the Beck Institute for Cognitive Therapy and Research and coauthor of *Think Confident, Be Confident.*

"That may sound difficult, but it's actually a simple matter of repetition," Dr. Sokol says. "If you think something again and again—like 'I'm my first priority'—and shift your behavior to reinforce that thought, it becomes ingrained, replacing unwanted habits in the process."

We asked three women to try this behavior shift by identifying a problematic trait, then following our expert-devised plans for change. Here you'll learn how it boosted their happiness—and what it could do for you. Change can be good!

THE OLD ME WAS TOO SHY!

LaNorma Huggins-Hopes, 44, married and a jewelry boutique owner in Woodbridge, Virginia

"I'm ultraconfident about the jewelry I design: It's my passion, and I know I'm good at it," Huggins-Hopes says. "But that's where my self-assurance ends. When it comes to mingling at networking events or meeting new people at a friend's get-together, I feel out of my comfort zone. I want to be able to initiate a conversation instead of waiting for people to come to me, and actively promote myself rather than just handing over my business card. I'm tired of letting my jewelry speak for me; I want to learn to express myself in a way that's as vibrant as my work!"

The Empowerment Plan

From Dr. Sokol: "LaNorma knows she's skilled as an artist but fails to acknowledge the amazing things she has to offer as a person. I think her shyness stems from a lack of experience with being bold. Once she practices self-assurance on a daily basis, it will begin to feel natural."

Make "so what?" your mantra. "Shyness comes from a fear of rejection or failure. Yes, you might stumble on occasion, and not everyone will be interested in you or your jewelry, but you're already a success, so who cares? Whenever you start to feel your self-doubts creeping in, ask yourself, 'So what?' And move forward."

Say something daring every day. "To feel confident, you'll have to act confident until it seems normal. With this in mind, every day, initiate a conversation with a stranger, solicit jewelry sales from a new client, or promote your work in person or on the phone. Don't worry about sounding good; the goal isn't to do it perfectly. It's just to do it."

Shrug off mistakes. "Focusing on the outcome rather than the process leads to fear, which inhibits confidence. To gain courage, try at least two new pursuits (go rock climbing, take a new art class, etc.) in which you're likely to make beginner's mistakes. Giving yourself permission to screw up will make the experience more fun and confidence-boosting."

The New Me

"Who knew it could be so easy to break out of my shell?" Huggins-Hopes says. "After the month, I felt downright bold! I've done things I never would have before: mingling at parties, cohosting events, even striking up conversations with strangers! When I feel my old self-doubt creep in, I get through it with the 'so what' mantra. To my surprise, I love saying something daring every day. So far I've contacted a designer to ask if she'd feature my jewelry in a show (she said yes!) and invited other fashion professionals to be on my blog. I've finally realized fear was my worst enemy, and rejection is better than never trying at all. Now I'm able to appreciate my successes and see myself as I see my jewelry: beautiful, colorful, and unique."

THE OLD ME WAS TOO NEGATIVE!

Mary K. Talbot, 47, married, mother of two boys ages 5 and 8, and a PR consultant in Barrington, Rhode Island

"I have a blessed life: wonderful children, a flexible career, and good health," Talbot says. "Still, I tend to focus on the negative more than I should. Perhaps it's because of the hardships I've encountered. My first child passed away 9 years ago, which naturally strained my marriage, and I've lost that 'glass is half full' feeling. This year, I started having digestive issues that my doctors can't explain, and I believe my negativity has something to do with it. I want to be a more positive person whom people want to be around, and I'm willing to put the work in to change my attitude."

The Optimism Plan

From Dr. Sokol: "The hardships Mary has dealt with have dampened her sense of optimism, but a few simple changes throughout her day will help her reshift her focus so she's able to keep her eyes on life's joys."

Practice mindfulness. "Chronic judgmental thoughts like 'I have to' or 'I should have' keep you from enjoying the current moment, which makes it hard to feel positive. When these thoughts strike, tell yourself, 'I'm here now,' and use your senses to be fully in the present."

Take a "silly break." "Print out a small monthly calendar. Your goal: Make two checkmarks daily—one for each time you were lighthearted, like humming, making a joke, or reading and acting out a character from one of your children's books. Adding a little levity will improve both your mood and that of those around you."

Put yourself first. "Putting your needs behind those of others can make you feel overwhelmed, which breeds negativity. Say no to requests or obligations at least twice a week. Say yes to your own needs by exercising, eating well, and sleeping 7 to 8 hours a night (even if you have to make compromises to do it). Once you make your well-being a priority, you'll feel better physically, which will help you maintain a positive attitude."

The New Me

"It's amazing that subtle changes made such a difference," Talbot says. "My stomach problems have eased up, and I'm better able to handle tense situations. For example, I recently ran into a woman who'd started a rumor about me, but I tuned her out and focused on being present with my son—seeing his smile turned my hurt feelings into joy. Interestingly, the best tip was the most obvious: Start sleeping. Getting 7 or 8 hours has meant letting my house go a bit, but the improvement in my mood has been worth it. Plus, my kids love the new me! They recently got soaked in a water gun fight and asked if they could run around in their underwear. They were shocked when I said yes, but it's so much easier to go with the flow."

THE OLD ME WAS A WORRYWART!

Natalie Mines, 44, married, mother of two boys ages 11 and 12, and a medical PR consultant on Long Island, New York

"Over the past year, I've become more forgetful," Mines says. "For example, another mom called to ask if my son was coming to her son's birthday party, which had started half an hour earlier! I'm always sending myself BlackBerry messages so I'll remember important stuff. I went to a neurologist, and tests revealed that my brain was in great shape, but the doctor said anxiety was making me operate at a less-than-optimal level. Trouble is, I've got something going from the minute I get up until I crawl in bed. I'm always stressed, and I snap in conflicts. But if I take time for myself, it makes me more anxious because of everything that needs to get done. I want to be calmer."

The Calming Plan

From expert Bruce Rabin, MD, PhD, medical director of the University of Pittsburgh Medical Center Healthy Lifestyle Program: "If your brain thinks it has to 'go' nonstop, it'll shift into emergency mode and shut down anyway. That's part of the reason stress leads to memory issues and exhaustion. To defuse her anxiety, Natalie needs to slow down and take care of herself."

Take a time-out. "Set aside a minimum of 10 minutes to do something relaxing—such as a short walk or some simple stretches—by 1:00 p.m. every day. At least once a week, allow yourself to reach a deeper state of relaxation by doing a meditation."

Write it down. "Anxiety stems from negative thoughts, which we're often not even aware of. To uncover and move past them, take 15 minutes once a week and write down what's on your mind. Even if it conjures some negative emotions, it could fuel helpful revelations. When you're done, rip the paper up. It's symbolic and will help you be honest, knowing no one will see it."

Acknowledge your influence on your kids. "As Natalie sensed, when you're tense, your children learn to mirror that behavior. Realizing this often leads to a breakthrough for moms, because even if you can't make your own wellness a priority, you'll do it for your kids."

The New Me

"I still have stress (who doesn't?), but now I have the tools to cope," Mines says. "I no longer snap in heated situations; instead, I calm down and deal. For example, my husband and I were having a tense conversation one night, but I defused it by saying, 'Let's talk tomorrow.' We ended up finding a good resolution. The writing exercise was a watershed for me. I realized certain people were causing me anxiety, which gave me strength to say 'Enough.' Since I started meditating, my house is running smoother, my kids are happier, and I'm less scattered at work. And yes, my memory is much better. This program has given me a new calm and opened my eyes to so many opportunities for joy."

CHAPTER 26

The Wisdom of Your Gut

It's smarter than you know, playing a significant role in mood, immunity, and intuition, and even keeping your skeleton strong. Here's how it's helping you right now— and how to further harness its extraordinary healing powers

Your gut: It's your second brain. Your gut is intimately involved in some intensely emotional business: We rely upon our gut instinct to tell us the right thing to do. We have a gut reaction to people who offend or delight us. We do a gut check when facing a challenge and congratulate ourselves when we display the intestinal fortitude, or guts, to take it on.

When you think about it, you won't be surprised to learn that your second brain is synced with your real brain. Just think about how a bout of intense fear or panic can liquefy your innards—or, more commonly, when a cramp or brief wave of nausea alerts you to a nagging anxiety your mind had been working so hard to suppress. There's a good reason your gut and your "first brain" communicate so seamlessly: Every class of neurochemical produced in the first brain is also produced in the second.

Another kind of chemical is the primary go-between for these two brains: stress hormones. When the brain detects any kind of threat—whether an impending layoff or a dustup with your spouse—it shoots stress hormones to your gut. Sensory nerves there respond by adjusting acid secretion and shutting down both appetite and digestion—a throwback to more dangerous times in our past, when we needed to summon all our resources to stand and fight, or flee. The result may be a nagging stomachache or a full-blown bout of GI distress.

Tummy trouble is the body's way of saying, "Pay attention to what's bugging you!" says clinical nutritionist Elizabeth Lipski, PhD, CCN, author of *Digestive Wellness* and *Digestive Wellness for Children.* "If my gut doesn't feel right, my job is to figure out what's out of balance." Although resolving work or personal problems requires long-term strategizing, you can tamp down the symptoms of a troubled gut with these tried-and-true anxiety-reducing techniques.

Breathe into your belly. Meditation, yoga, deep breathing, and other practices that encourage mindful relaxation make the body less sensitive to stress, research suggests. Deep breathing, using the muscles of your diaphragm (you should feel your belly expand and deflate with each inhale and exhale), can also help calm your mind and release tension in your abdominal muscles, easing indigestion. Another way to calm the body's autonomic nervous system—which regulates digestion, among other things—is through progressive muscle relaxation, tightening and then relaxing small groups of muscles beginning in your toes and working your way up to your face.

Go for easy workouts. Moderate exercise is a known enemy of stress. (Whenever you can, exercise outdoors. Natural settings help calm frayed nerves.) Start slowly and increase activity gradually. Even a 20-minute stroll will help soothe nerves, improve digestion, and reduce bloating, gas, and constipation by optimizing the passage of waste through your bowels.

Remember: Your ultimate goal in soothing a troubled tummy is to get clearer intuitive signals. When something really bugs you, your second brain will let you know loud and clear.

YOUR GUT IS ALSO A FUEL REFINERY

Once you've polished off a meal, you probably don't give it much thought. But when you push away from the table, your gut's work is only beginning. It will take between 9 hours and a day or two for the food you just ate to be fully digested. During that time, your stomach and small intestine break your food down into molecules that the small intestine's thin lining can absorb, allowing essential nutrients—the energy stream that fuels every cell in your body—to enter your bloodstream. The lower part of your small intestine then wrings out the water remaining in your meal and ushers it into your colon, which funnels it into your bloodstream to help keep you hydrated.

As straightforward as this process sounds, the seemingly simple chore of digestion depends on a finely orchestrated series of muscular contractions, chemical secretions, and electrical signals all along the 30-foot-long gastrointestinal tract. But there's also plenty you can do to keep this operation running smoothly.

Follow its pace. A rushed meal is out of sync with the creeping pace of the gut. Savor your meal. In a neat bit of mind/body magic, the thought, sight, and aroma of good food jump-start the digestive process, signaling the stomach and salivary glands to secrete chemicals that will help break down food. Chew your food well so your gut doesn't have to work as hard to break it down. Eat slowly to avoid gulping air, which will make you gassy, bloated, and—thanks to the mind's payback to the body—irritable.

Nurture its residents. Gut-friendly bacteria use fiber, an indigestible carbohydrate, as their main food source, so eat plenty of fruits, vegetables, and whole grains such as oats, barley, whole wheat, and popcorn. Fiber also aids the passage of food and waste through the gut. Most adult women should aim for over 20 grams of fiber a day; men should get at least 30 grams. But again, go slowly: Increasing your fiber intake too quickly can cause gas and bloating.

Respect its opinions. Even the most finely tuned machine has its quirks. If certain foods trigger GI problems for you, avoid them. Common heartburn culprits include acidic, spicy, and fatty foods; caffeinated and carbonated drinks; chocolate; and onions. Notorious gas producers include beans, onions, and cruciferous vegetables such as cauliflower, cabbage, and radishes. (These veggies are loaded with vital nutrients, so don't shun them altogether, but enjoy them in small doses.) The same goes for packaged low-carb treats and other foods containing artificial sweeteners—especially the sweetener sorbitol.

Lighten its load. People who are overweight are more likely to suffer from GI problems. Whatever your weight, though, regular exercise can help alleviate digestive distress. In a study involving 983 people participating in a weight-loss program, the more physical activity people got each week, the fewer GI symptoms they had. Aim for at least 20 minutes of moderate activity each day.

YOUR GUT IS ALSO YOUR SHIELD AGAINST GERMS

If you've ever had food poisoning, you know your gut is an uncompromising vigilante. When a nasty microbe hitchhikes a ride into the body on the back of real food, the gut quickly recognizes the interloper and strong-arms it to the nearest exit. To make the ID in the first place, it calls upon a reliable army of sentries, millions of immune system cells residing in its walls.

If the fact that the gut plays a major role in immunity sounds surprising, consider that the whole purpose of the immune system is to differentiate what's you from what's not you. Then consider that every day, you introduce pounds of foreign material—your daily bread—into your gut. The immune system has to decide what's okay to let through and what's not, so it makes sense to headquarter that process right where the food comes in.

This powerful system gears up from day 1. A newborn's gastrointestinal tract is entirely germ free, but immediately after birth, pioneering bacteria begin to colonize it. In the first few years of life, everyone's gut develops a unique extended family of bacterial species, determined in part by genetics and in part by diet, hygiene, medication use, and the bacteria colonizing those around us. Perhaps bacteria's most important job: stimulating and training the body's immune system and, by their overwhelming presence, crowding out more harmful critters.

The specific microbial mix (your gut contains thousands of species of bacteria) you wind up with has a big impact on your health. Besides making you more resistant to disease, the balance (or lack thereof) of microbes in your gut may lower your risk of obesity or influence your risk of autoimmune disorders such as rheumatoid arthritis, multiple sclerosis, psoriasis, and inflammatory bowel disease. Clearly, this extended family deserves coddling. Here are immune-boosting ways to protect it.

Steer clear of detoxes. Colonic "cleanses" rid the colon of good bacteria and can cause overgrowth of bad bacteria.

Avoid overusing antibiotics. They kill not only pathogens causing your ailment but also good bacteria.

Consume foods with probiotics. Look for yogurts and soy milks that contain strains of *Lactobacillus* and *Bifidobacteria*. In addition to protecting against colds and flu and promoting healthful bacteria, probiotics can help relieve diarrhea caused by infection or antibiotics, irritable bowel syndrome, or Crohn's disease.

CHAPTER 27

Field of Dreams

Sleep cures are not one-size-fits-all. Here are dozens of pillow-tested, all-natural, sound-sleep secrets tailored to your nightly needs to help you sleep better tonight—and feel better tomorrow

Sound slumber results in increased energy and productivity, improved heart and immune system health, a better mood, even a longer life. And hey, you just feel so much better after a satisfying 8 hours of rest. But chances are, you're not getting it. "Sleep issues are epidemic today," says Michael Breus, PhD, clinical psychologist and author of *The Sleep Doctor's Diet Plan*.

Not surprisingly, women tend to get less sleep than men do overall, says Marianne Legato, MD, director of the Partnership for Gender-Specific Medicine at Columbia University. Pregnancy can keep a woman up; along with the hormonal imbalances, she might lie awake with gastroesophageal reflux disease (GERD) and nasal congestion. There's the staggering lack of postpregnancy sleep, too. Even if women don't have children, levels of sleep-promoting estrogen sink regularly during menstruation and then permanently in

GATHER A DREAM GROUP

Book groups? Been there, done that. The newest trend is dream groups, in which a "dream worker" or therapist leads a discussion to interpret a dream. The process solders a profound bond. "We offer feedback on each other's emotional blind spots," says Anne Hill, who is a member of such a club in Sebastopol, California. Here's how to start your own group.

GATHER A FEW FRIENDS. Choose friends who know each other well—enough to get a good discussion going. Five to nine people seems to be ideal.

ESTABLISH A TIME LIMIT. This gives each participant time to share her dreams and receive feedback.

KEEP DISCUSSIONS CONFIDENTIAL. "This is soul work, and our souls are deeply vulnerable," advises Diana McKendree of the Haden Institute of Flat Rock, North Carolina.

GIVE IT A TRIAL RUN. Take 4 weeks to check out the group's dynamics. If everyone's happy, keep going.

menopause. And symptoms related to both—cramps, headaches, hot flashes, and night sweats—also disrupt slumber. Nor does the situation improve with age: Older women need midnight bathroom breaks more often than men do, says Dr. Legato, and anxiety (which likewise rises with age) also causes—you guessed it—sleep problems.

But experts agree that these biological facts don't mean that sleep deprivation has to be a woman's destiny. "Feeling tired should never be considered normal," says Dr. Breus. Yet there are no stock sleep solutions, either: Finding out what works for you takes some trial and error, but it's well worth it, says Lawrence Epstein, MD, chief medical officer of Sleep HealthCenters. "Sleep is a basic biological necessity—just like eating—and it has an impact on every aspect of your health and your life," he notes.

We've taken the top three sleeping-problem patterns—trouble falling asleep, trouble staying asleep, and awakening easily (see explanations of each of these below in "What's Your Sleep Struggle")—and highlighted the best natural solutions for each. Use them to customize your personal plan for getting the rest you need—starting tonight.

WHAT'S YOUR SLEEP STRUGGLE?

Sleep challenges fall into the following three categories. Once you identify yours, you can tailor the tips to yourself.

"I Can't Fall Asleep"

No matter how hard you try to will yourself into dreamland, you toss, turn, and remain frustrated and wide awake. Your mind may be racing through tomorrow's daunting to-do list, only to realize how much more impossible it will all be if you can't get to sleep—right now! That ruminating, of course, only keeps you even more firmly awake in a snarled circle of sleeplessness and stress.

"I Can't Stay Asleep"

It's 3:00 a.m., and suddenly your eyes pop open, like they do pretty much every night at this hour. You alternate between watching the clock and staring at your sleeping husband's back, resenting them both equally. Maybe you get up for a little while, maybe you just lie there, but finally you doze off—and the alarm rings what seems like seconds later.

"Every Little Thing Wakes Me Up"

You fall right asleep, but you're supersensitive to your environment, and as soon as you close your eyes, something jolts you awake, again and again. Maybe it's the light from your clock radio; maybe it's a branch scraping against the window; maybe your pillow is too flat, your room is too warm, or your socks are too tight.

TO NAP OR NOT TO NAP?

That is the question when you're drowsy after lunch, but the answer is that, well, it depends. In the afternoon, your energy levels are likely to dip naturally, and napping can improve alertness, performance, and memory. So if you're sleep deprived and circumstances allow, indulge! Your nap should start before 3:00 p.m. and last 30 minutes or less—otherwise your body may enter a deep-sleep phase, which means you'll feel groggy when you wake. If you can't nap, try a quick brisk walk to refresh yourself.

STICK WITH A CONSISTENT SLEEP SCHEDULE

Try it if you can't fall asleep.

If you do only one thing to improve your sleep, this is it, says Dr. Breus: Go to bed at the same time every night and get up at the same time every morning—even on weekends. A regular sleep routine keeps your biological clock steady so you rest better. Exposure to a regular pattern of light and dark helps, so stay in sync by opening the blinds or going outside right after you wake up.

KEEP A SLEEP DIARY

Try it if you can't fall asleep or if you awaken easily.

To help you understand how your habits affect your rest, track your sleep every day for at least 2 weeks. Write down not only what's obviously sleep related—what time you go to bed, how long it takes you to fall asleep, how many times you wake up during the night, how you feel in the morning—but also factors like what you ate close to bedtime and what exercise you got. Comparing your daily activities with your nightly sleep patterns can show you where you need to make changes. For a sample sleep diary, go to www.sleepdoctor.com.

STOP SMOKING

Try it if you can't fall asleep, can't stay asleep, or awaken easily.

Reason number 1,001 to quit: Nicotine is a stimulant, so it prevents you from falling asleep. Plus, many smokers experience withdrawal pangs at night. Smokers are four times more likely not to feel as well rested after a night's sleep than nonsmokers, studies show, and smoking exacerbates sleep apnea and other breathing disorders, which can also stop you from getting a good night's rest.

Don't worry that quitting will keep you up nights, too: That effect passes in about 3 nights, says Lisa Shives, MD, sleep expert and founder of North-shore Sleep Medicine.

REVIEW YOUR MEDICATIONS

Try it if you can't fall asleep or you awaken easily.

Beta blockers (prescribed for high blood pressure) may cause insomnia; so can SSRIs (a class of antidepressants that includes Prozac and Zoloft). And that's just the beginning. Write down every drug and supplement you take, and have your doctor evaluate how they may be affecting your sleep.

WHEN IS YOUR BEST BEDTIME?

Most people need between 7 and 9 hours of sleep per night, but one size really doesn't fit all when it comes to slumber. To find out what will work best for you, take your normal wake-up time, then count backward 7½ hours to determine when to hit the sack. That means if your morning typically starts at 6:00 a.m., you should be in bed by 10:30 p.m. If you wake up a few minutes before your alarm goes off, bingo! You've found your perfect bedtime. If you were still fast asleep, try hitting the hay 20 minutes earlier each night until you find the time that works for you.

EXERCISE, BUT NOT WITHIN 4 HOURS OF BEDTIME

Try it if you can't fall asleep.

Working out—especially cardio—improves the length and quality of your sleep, says Dr. Shives. That said, 30 minutes of vigorous aerobic exercise keeps your body temperature elevated for about 4 hours, inhibiting sleep. When your body begins to cool down, however, it signals your brain to release sleep-inducing melatonin, so then you'll get drowsy.

CUT CAFFEINE AFTER 2:00 P.M.

Try it if you can't fall asleep or if you can't stay asleep.

That means coffee, tea, and cola. Caffeine is a stimulant that stays in your system for about 8 hours, so if you have a cappuccino after dinner, come bedtime, it'll either prevent your brain from entering deep sleep or stop you from falling asleep altogether.

"WHEN I SLEEP LATE TO CATCH UP, I FEEL WORSE. WHY?"

Probably because even with those extra hours, you still haven't made up for your total cumulative sleep deficit. Here's the math: Say you need 8 hours of solid slumber every night, but during a particularly hectic workweek, you got only 6. You owe your "sleep bank" the full 10 hours you've missed. If you sleep late on the weekend to try to catch up, you won't feel refreshed, because your body will slip into sounder sleep in an attempt to compensate for that shortfall of hours. That means that when you get up after just an extra hour or two, your body has to pull itself out of a profoundly deep level of sleep, which can leave you feeling more wiped out than ever.

So what's the best way to pay back your sleep debt? Go to bed just slightly earlier than usual for several nights in a row; that won't throw off your body clock as much.

67

THE PERCENTAGE OF AMERICAN WOMEN
WHO SAY THEY FREQUENTLY HAVE
PROBLEMS SLEEPING

WRITE DOWN YOUR WOES

Try it if you can't fall asleep.

"The number-one sleep complaint I hear? 'I can't turn off my mind,'" says Dr. Breus. To quiet that wakeful worrying, every night jot down your top concerns—say, I have to call my insurer to dispute that denied claim, which will take forever, and how can I spend all that time on the phone when work is so busy? Then write down the steps you can take to solve the problem—I'm going to look up the numbers before breakfast, refuse to stay on hold for more than 3 minutes, and send e-mails tomorrow night if I can't get through. Or even, I can't do anything about this tonight, so I'll worry about it tomorrow.

Once your concerns are converted into some kind of action plan, you'll rest easier.

TAKE TIME TO WIND DOWN

Try it if you can't fall asleep or can't stay asleep.

"Sleep is not an on-off switch," says Dr. Breus. "It's more like slowly easing your foot off the gas." Give your body time to transition from your active day to bedtime drowsiness by setting a timer for an hour before bed and divvying up the time as follows:

First 20 minutes: Prep for tomorrow (pack your bag, set out your clothes).

Next 20: Take care of personal hygiene (brush your teeth, moisturize your face).

Last 20: Relax in bed, reading by a small, low-wattage book light or practicing deep breathing.

SIP MILK, NOT A MARTINI

Try it if you can't stay asleep.

A few hours after you drink, alcohol levels in your blood start to drop, which signals your body to wake up. It takes an average person about an hour to metabolize one drink, so if you have two glasses of wine with dinner, finish your last sip at least 2 hours before bed.

SNACK ON CHEESE AND CRACKERS

Try it if you can't fall asleep.

The ideal nighttime nosh combines carbohydrates and either calcium or a protein that contains the amino acid tryptophan. Studies show that both of these combos boost serotonin, a naturally occurring brain chemical that helps you feel calm. Enjoy your snack about an hour before bedtime so that the amino acids have time to reach your brain.

Some good choices: one piece of whole grain toast with a slice of low-fat cheese or turkey, a banana with 1 teaspoon of peanut butter, whole grain cereal and fat-free milk, or fruit and low-fat yogurt.

LISTEN TO A BEDTIME STORY

Try it if you can't fall asleep.

Load a familiar audiobook on your iPod—one that you know well, so it doesn't engage you but distracts your attention until you drift off to sleep, suggests Dr. Shives. Relaxing music works well, too.

STAY COOL

Try it if you can't fall asleep or can't stay asleep.

Experts usually recommend setting your bedroom thermostat between 65° and 75°F, which is a good guideline, but pay attention to how you actually

SIDE EFFECTS OF SLEEP DEPRIVATION

Sleep deprivation is often the fodder for sit-com jokes. But fatigue is really no laughing matter. Here's why.

After just 1 night of poor sleep . . .

- Your skin suffers. You look pasty and ashen, and under-eye circles grow darker and deeper.
- You make bad decisions. Your prefrontal cortex—the part of your brain that controls logic—shuts down, so you may make mistakes.
- Your muscles hurt. Sleeplessness depletes serotonin and increases pain sensitivity.
- You're cranky. Being tired leads to irritability and increased anxiety.

After a few nights . . .

- You can't concentrate. Or focus. Or complete simple tasks. Or even remember what tasks you wanted to complete. Consistently getting only a few hours of sleep a night may affect you just as much as not being able to sleep at all.
- You increase your risk of diabetes. Losing just 3 to 4 hours of sleep over several days reduces your ability to keep blood sugar levels on an even keel.

Long-term sleep loss leads to . . .

OBESITY: Too little sleep triggers metabolic changes that cause you to store fat more easily.

HEART DISEASE: Without rest, your heart muscle is overworked, which can cause high blood pressure or thickening of the heart muscle.

PSYCHOLOGICAL DISTURBANCES: Poor sleep can cause mood swings and is linked with depression.

REDUCED IMMUNITY: Your immune system can't work at capacity.

feel under the covers. Slipping between cool sheets helps trigger a drop in your body temperature. That shift signals the body to produce melatonin, which induces sleep.

That's why it's also a good idea to take a warm bath or hot shower before going to bed: Both temporarily raise your body temperature, after which it gradually lowers in the cooler air, cueing your body to feel sleepy. But for optimal rest, once you've settled in to bed, you shouldn't feel cold or hot—but just right.

SET THE THERMOSTAT EVEN LOWER

Try it if you can't stay asleep or if you awaken easily.

During menopause, 75 percent of women suffer from hot flashes, and just over 20 percent have night sweats or hot flashes that trouble their sleep. Consider turning on a fan or the AC to cool and circulate the air. Just go low gradually: Your body loses some ability to regulate its temperature during rapid eye movement (REM) sleep, so overchilling your environment—down to 60°F, for instance—will backfire.

Try this tip even if you're not menopausal.

INFUSE YOUR ROOM WITH A SLEEP-INDUCING SCENT

Try it if you can't fall asleep.

Certain smells, such as lavender, chamomile, and ylang-ylang, activate the alpha wave activity in the back of your brain, which leads to relaxation and helps you sleep more soundly. Mix a few drops of essential oil and water in a spray bottle and give your pillowcase a spritz.

TURN ON WHITE NOISE

Try it if you awaken easily.

Sound machines designed to help you sleep produce a low-level soothing noise. These can help you tune out barking dogs, the TV downstairs, or any other disturbances so you can fall asleep and stay asleep.

ELIMINATE LIGHT SOURCES

Try it if you can't stay asleep or if you awaken easily.

"Light is a powerful signal to your brain to be awake," explains Dr. Shives. Even the glow from your laptop, iPad, smartphone, or any other electronics on your nightstand may pass through your closed eyelids and retinas into your hypothalamus—the part of your brain that controls sleep. This delays your brain's release of the sleep-promoting hormone melatonin. Thus, the darker your room is, the more soundly you'll sleep.

CONSIDER KICKING OUT FURRY BEDMATES

Try it if you awaken easily.

Cats can be active in the late-night and early morning hours, and dogs may scratch, sniff, and snore you awake. More than half of people who sleep with their pets say the animals disturb their slumber, according to a survey from the Mayo Clinic Sleep Disorders Center.

"But if your pet is a good, sound sleeper and snuggling up with him is comforting and soothing, it's fine to let him stay put," advises Dr. Shives.

CHECK YOUR PILLOW POSITION

Try it if you awaken easily.

The perfect prop for your head will keep your spine and neck in a straight line to avoid tension or cramps that can prevent you from falling asleep. Ask your spouse to check the alignment of your head and neck when you're in your starting sleep position. If your neck is flexed back or raised, get a pillow that lets you sleep in a better-aligned position. And if you're a stomach sleeper, consider using either no pillow or a very flat one to help keep your neck and spine straight.

BREATHE—DEEPLY

Try it if you can't fall asleep or if you can't stay asleep.

This technique helps reduce your heart rate and blood pressure, releases endorphins, and relaxes your body, priming you for sleep. Inhale for 5 seconds,

DREAM ON!

Dreams are finally getting the respect they deserve, as pathways that illuminate our deepest desires, fears, and frustrations. Better yet, they can actually give us the courage and confidence to act.

Jan Brehm of Portland woke up from a dream confused and shaken to her core. Lisa Espich of Tucson woke so deeply disturbed by a dream featuring her husband that she knew her marriage would never be the same. Jennifer Lambert of Virginia Beach felt such agitation over her dream that she cried for 30 minutes straight when she woke up—and then called her sister, from whom she'd long been estranged.

Dreams can rock us, scare us, and in some cases, inspire us. But is listening to our dreams right up there with calling a psychic hotline? Not at all, say leading experts. "People are now using their dreams as tools to make their lives better," comments Marcia Emery, PhD, a psychologist at Holos University.

This is relatively newfound respect. Many researchers used to believe that dreams simply reflected the random firing of nerve signals while we sleep. "The thinking was that the dreams were meaningless and didn't serve any function at all," says Harvard psychology professor Deirdre Barrett, PhD. But today, many scientists feel that dreams play the vital role of clarifying what truly matters to us. "Dreaming is thinking—just in a different biochemical state," explains Dr. Barrett, author of *The Committee of Sleep: How Artists, Scientists, and Athletes Use Dreams for Creative Problem-Solving—and How You Can Too.* "It's a mode of contemplation that's much more visual, intuitive, and emotional, as opposed to the patterns of waking thought."

It's that intuitiveness that makes so-called "epiphany" dreams such a valuable resource. "Dreams can provide inspiration or help you get unstuck from problems because your mind is working on things in this different way," Dr. Barrett says. Case in point: When she gave subjects instruction in a technique called "dream incubation," half of them dreamed about a problem they had focused on prior to going to sleep, and a full 25 percent had a dream that provided an actionable solution.

Granted, listening to the dreaming brain isn't easy. "Even though it might feel like it's a bizarre, cryptic language, if you can decode it, what remains is brutal self-honesty," explains Lauri Quinn Loewenberg, a member of the International Association for the Study of Dreams and founder of TheDreamZone.com. "When you start connecting dreams with your waking life, you're able to see yourself and your true inner thoughts much more clearly."

Finding the meaning in your dreams is like growing a garden, the pros say: The more you do it, the greater the insights it yields. "If you're regularly tending your dreams, once in a while you'll have a breakthrough that grabs you by the throat," Dr. Barrett says. Here are three women whose dreams provided just such revelations.

Jan Brehm, 56, an Actress with Two Daughters, in Portland, Oregon

THE DREAM: "I went into the bathroom and pulled back the shower curtain. There was my daughter, now 26, at age 10 months. I felt a wave of horror. She was sitting in the tub shivering, and her lips were blue. I had forgotten I'd left her there. When I woke up, I was so disturbed that I couldn't shake off the image."

WHAT IT MEANS: According to Loewenberg: "When you dream about someone very close to you, human nature is to figure out if the dream is literally about that person. But it may instead represent some part of your current life. I asked Jan what was going on with her daughter: Was there any guilt she was feeling? Jan said that was not the case, which was why the dream scared her so deeply.

"Since there didn't seem to be an issue with her daughter, I suggested that the infant might symbolize something else in her life that she'd been neglecting. We often refer to our ventures and projects as 'our baby,' because, like a baby, they are things that we must nourish and care for so they can reach their potential.

"You might not expect such a frightening dream to be associated with something joyful. But Jan's dreaming mind chose to send the message through a strong negative emotion in order to grab her attention."

WHAT SHE DID: "Several years back, I'd started to write and produce a DVD series on menopause, but when I couldn't get the funding for it, I stopped working on it," says Jan. "So when Lauri asked me if I had a creative project that I had abandoned, it stopped me cold. I knew instantly that the shivering baby was the menopause

(continued)

series. I plunged myself into the work, and I launched the DVD 2 years ago. The dream gave me the impetus to move forward."

Lisa Spich, 41, Married to a Man with a Drug Dependence, in Tucson, Arizona

THE DREAM: "I woke in the middle of the night to find my husband was not in bed. I could hear a loud buzzing sound, so I got up to investigate. When I looked out into the backyard, I could see a spotlight hanging down from a tree. Under the light, I could see that my husband had set up a table saw. As I got closer, I could make out a woman's bloody torso. Several of her limbs were scattered on the ground.

"I noticed that our neighbor was looking over the fence and I knew that he would be calling the police. I panicked and told my husband that we needed to hide the body. I helped him dig a hole to bury the woman's remains. As we dug up the dirt, however, other limbs and body parts started to come to the surface. Soon our yard was filled with the remains of these other women. We finished burying the last of the evidence just before the sound of police sirens filled the air. When I answered the door, I acted as if everything was perfectly fine, but the police gave me a truth serum to get me to talk. As soon as I took it, the truth came out. When I woke up, I was sick to my stomach. I couldn't even talk to my husband."

WHAT IT MEANS: According to Dr. Emery: "In the dream, Lisa has gone to investigate the situation, and the 'spotlight' is on her. As the dirt is dug up and the body parts start to surface, the facts are coming to light—that is, people are finding out about her husband's addiction.

"The biggest key turns when you take the word *kill* and associate it with similar words: such as *shoot, gun, murder.* The translation is that Lisa, the dreamer, is putting an end to the secrecy of her husband's addiction. To use an old cliché, the truth—represented by the truth serum in her dreams—will set her free."

WHAT SHE DID: "What really stuck with me from the dream was the sense of relief I felt once the truth came out," admits Lisa. "So I gathered the courage to do exactly what the dream was suggesting: I told my secret. Once my family knew the truth, they helped give me the strength to walk away from the situation.

"Amazingly, after I left, my husband was able to find his own courage and seek treatment for his addiction. He has now been clean and sober for more than 5 years, and our marriage is healthy again."

Jennifer Lambert, 35, Whose Grandfather Had Died 3 Weeks Earlier, in Virginia Beach, Virginia

THE DREAM: "My grandfather came to our house, and I was so excited to see him that I wrapped my arms around his neck for a hug. His first words were 'Don't be angry at your sister anymore.'

"At the time, my sister and I couldn't even be in the same room. While I'm the older one, she is definitely more aggressive, so I always held back what I thought for fear of her retaliating. When I woke up, I cried for about 30 minutes."

WHAT IT MEANS: According to Dr. Barrett: "Sometimes it takes a dream to 'see' our grief and sadness, like what Jennifer felt toward her sister. Dreams are more likely to let the more divergent feelings inside us rise to our consciousness.

"The timing—just 3 weeks after her grandfather's death—suggests that this loss may have stirred up feelings about someone else Jennifer was missing: her sister. Her grandfather is someone she associated with a loving attitude, and it's usually people with a particular trait whom we select in dreams to voice an aspect of ourselves that's getting shortchanged in waking life. It would be difficult to offer her sister an olive branch when their relationship appeared so deadlocked, but the dream gave a clear push in that direction."

WHAT SHE DID: "A few days after the dream, I spoke to my sister and told her that I didn't like the way our relationship was going," recalls Jennifer, "and that I wanted our connection to be more like our mom and our aunt, who were very close. We still had a few rocky spots after that conversation, but now we're best friends. I don't know if our reconciliation would have happened without that dream."

pause for 3, then exhale to a count of 5. Start with eight repetitions; gradually increase to 15.

To see if you're doing it right, says Dr. Breus, buy a bottle of children's bubbles, breathe in through your belly, and blow through the wand. The smooth and steady breath that you use to blow a bubble successfully should be what you strive for when you're trying to get to sleep.

STAY PUT IF YOU WAKE UP

Try it if you can't stay asleep or you awaken easily.

"The textbook advice is that if you can't fall back asleep in 15 minutes, get out of bed," says Dr. Shives. "But I ask my patients, 'How do you feel in bed?' If they're not fretting or anxious, I tell them to stay there, in the dark, and do some deep breathing or visualization." But if lying in bed pushes your stress buttons, get up and do something quiet and relaxing (in dim light), such as gentle yoga or massaging your feet, until you feel sleepy again.

WAGING WAR ON ALZHEIMER'S

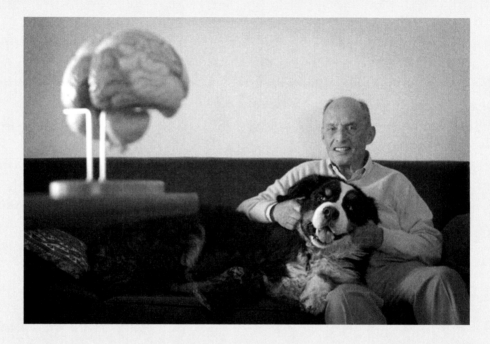

In 1948, when Paul Greengard was just 23, he hit a career crossroads that involved a stark moral choice. He wanted to earn a degree in theoretical physics, but the only fellowships were funded by the Atomic Energy Commission. Unwilling to contribute to weapons of mass destruction, he instead decided to concentrate on the new field of biophysics, earning a doctorate from Johns Hopkins University.

His choice may benefit millions of people who develop Alzheimer's disease. Dr. Greengard first studied nerve cell communication, which led to the development of antidepressants such as Prozac, and in 2000, he was awarded the Nobel Prize for his research. Then, about 15 years ago, at an age when others are long retired, he turned his focus to Alzheimer's after watching his father-in-law suffer from it.

"I knew this was something worthwhile," says Dr. Greengard, 84, who still works 7 days a week in his lab at Rockefeller University.

Worthwhile, indeed. His lab recently announced an Alzheimer's breakthrough that might one day lead to a cure. The main culprit in the disease is thought to be an excess of beta-amyloid, a protein that clumps in the brain, interfering with crucial functions. Dr. Greengard's team identified the specific enzyme (named gSAP) that triggers that overproduction. A drug that disables that enzyme may one day end Alzheimer's. He hopes that clinical trials start within 3 years, and a cure could get to market within 6 to 10.

Dr. Greengard is also a champion of women. The soft-spoken scientist used the $400,000 he received for his Nobel Prize (along with other prize money and his own funds) to start a $50,000 yearly award to recognize women scientists, named for his mother: the Pearl Meister Greengard Prize. Today, women still face discrimination in science, and Dr. Greengard hopes his award will help draw attention to their achievements.

One of the biggest roadblocks to a cure is a lack of patients to test new drugs. Now TrialMatch , from the nonprofit Alzheimer's Association, might help by pairing patients with clinical trials based on personal profiles they create. Encouraging someone you know to sign up could help end Alzheimer's sooner. Visit www.alz.org/trialmatch for details.

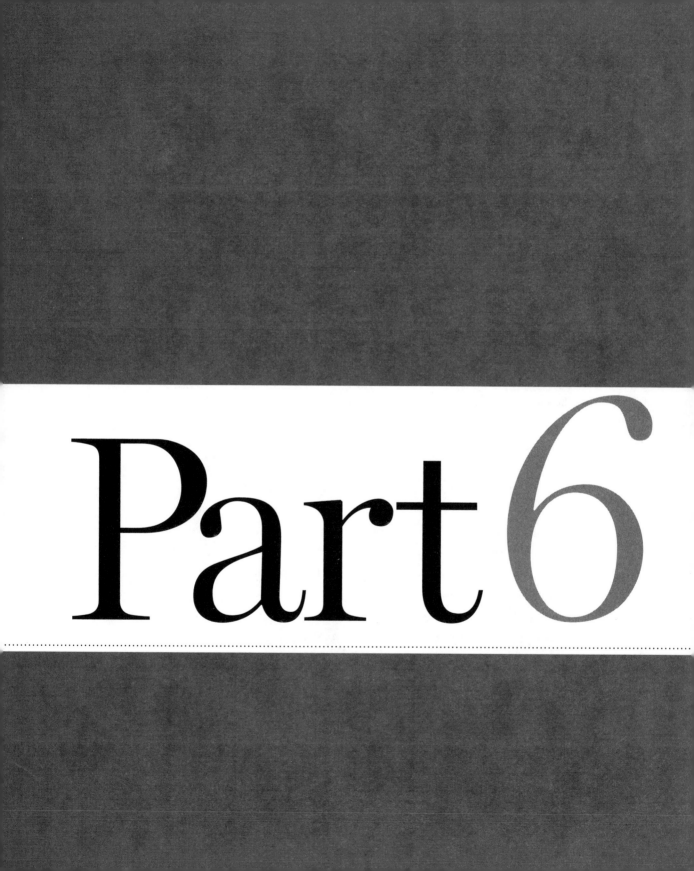

Part 6

BEAUTY
BREAKTHROUGHS

CHAPTER 28

The Age-Erasing Plan

No more skin excuses! Break these bad habits and take years off your complexion

Skipping sunscreen on a gray winter day or flopping into bed in makeup is unlikely to do any real harm, but too many lapses in beauty judgment could lead to signs of age. The flip side? Taking a few minutes a day for smart skin care can prevent years' worth of wrinkles, brown spots, and more. Whether you're a repeat offender or just make the occasional mistake, here are five common excuses that could be aging your skin, plus simple solutions to keep you looking young.

"IT'S BEEN A LONG DAY, AND THE LAST THING I WANT TO DO IS WASH MY FACE."

No more excuses: The 2 minutes it takes to cleanse before bed helps ensure a fresh-faced look for years. "Sleeping with dirt, oil, and makeup on causes acne and enlarged pores," says Audrey Kunin, MD, an associate clinical instructor of dermatology at the University of Kansas School of Medicine.

To easily remove debris, keep no-rinse face wipes in your nightstand.

Try: Boots No7 Quick Thinking 4-in-1 Wipes ($7; Target) or Pond's Clean Sweep Age Defying Wet Cleansing Towelettes ($6.50; CVS).

"I DON'T NEED SUNSCREEN, IT'S WINTER!"

No more excuses: Exposure to UVA rays, the primary culprit behind aging, happens all year long. And because they can penetrate glass, you're susceptible even when you're indoors, says Fredric Brandt, MD, a New York– and Miami-based dermatologist.

THREE SNEAKY ACNE CULPRITS

Long past puberty but still breaking out? Here are some possible unusual acne promoters.

TALC-CONTAINING POWDER MAKEUP. This mineral is made up of tiny crystals that can clog pores, says Macrene Alexiades-Armenakas, MD, PhD, assistant clinical professor of dermatology at Yale University School of Medicine. Instead, try Physicians Formula Mineral Wear Talc-Free Mineral Face Powder ($13; drugstores).

DAIRY. The biggest milk drinkers are more likely to experience breakouts, finds research, possibly because dairy products contain the same hormones that stimulate oil production in humans. It's not proven, but dermatologists report that eating cheese, yogurt, and ice cream also triggers acne. Give up all dairy for a few months to see if your skin clears. In the meantime, take a calcium supplement.

A LACK OF NATURAL OILS. Phytosphingosine, a type of fat that kills acne-causing bacteria and reduces inflammation, helps keep pores clear. To supplement skin's supply, try DermaDoctor Ain't Misbehavin' Intensive Skin-Correcting Sulfur Acne Mask ($45; www.dermadoctor.com).

FIVE SKIN OATHS YOU WON'T REGRET

Kudos to you! You're exercising and eating healthy. But to hit a health home run, pay attention to your skin. It's the body's largest organ, and it has an enormous effect on your psyche. (When your skin looks good, you feel good.) Bonus: Becoming intimately familiar with your skin might even save you from disease. Commit to the following changes.

I WILL TAKE CARE OF MY NECK. Like your face, your neck is vulnerable to UV damage. Protect it with sunscreen daily, along with your chest and hands.

I WILL NOT WASH WITH HOT WATER. High temps strip skin of its natural oils, causing dryness and irritation. If you don't want to give up hot showers, cleanse your face first with lukewarm water—and keep it out of the shower stream.

I WILL NOT EXERCISE WITH MAKEUP ON. Cosmetics and sweat clog pores more than does sweat alone, causing breakouts and enlarged pores.

I WILL GET AN ANNUAL FULL-BODY SKIN EXAM. See a dermatologist yearly to check for any moles that have changed color or texture or to examine other lesions that might signal skin cancer.

I WILL UPDATE MY BEAUTY PRODUCTS. Each product category has its own shelf life, based on its ingredients and preservatives.

Mascara: Replace every 6 months.

Sunscreen: It's usually effective for up to 3 years when stored correctly. (High temps render it ineffective.) Check the expiration date on the bottle.

Antiagers: Ingredients like retinoids and AHAs are effective for 3 months to a year. Antioxidants like vitamin C last about 6 months once opened.

The number one way to guard against this and keep skin looking youthful: Every day, use a sunscreen or moisturizer with an SPF 30 that's labeled broad-spectrum. For the best protection, choose one that contains either avobenzone, Helioplex, Mexoryl, titanium dioxide, or zinc oxide.

Try: Olay Professional Pro-x Age Repair Lotion with SPF 30 ($42; drugstores) or Aveeno Positively Ageless Daily Moisturizer, SPF 30 ($20; drugstores).

"TAKING CARE OF MY SKIN COSTS TOO MUCH MONEY."

No more excuses: To save, shop at drugstores. Studies show that mass products are as effective as (and sometimes more than!) pricier lines. "Look for active ingredients, not fancy labels," says David E. Bank, MD, an associate professor of dermatology at Columbia University/New York-Presbyterian Hospital.

The most effective antiagers include retinoids, AHAs, peptides, vitamin C, and hydrators such as hyaluronic acid.

"I'VE GIVEN UP. I'VE TRIED ALMOST EVERYTHING, AND NOTHING SEEMS TO WORK."

No more excuses: It can take at least 8 weeks to see the results of many ingredients, so give products time to deliver their benefits. Another must: Incorporate new products slowly—one about every 2 months.

"Your skin needs to build up a tolerance to aggressive antiagers," says Dr. Bank. "Going overboard can cause inflammation, which accelerates fine lines, brown spots, and sagging."

"EXFOLIATING MAKES MY FACE RED AND IRRITATED."

No more excuses: Getting rid of dead cells helps soften wrinkles and brighten skin, but aggressive scrubs can lead to redness and irritation. To slough safely, choose a chemical exfoliator, such as glycolic acid, or gentle cleansing beads. Avoid scrubs with an uneven texture, such as walnut shells.

Exfoliate just once or twice a week if you're using an OTC or Rx retinoid or AHA. It alone provides sufficient skin sloughing.

MYTHS THAT AGE YOUR SKIN

What you don't know—or think you do know—about your skin can sap its youthful luster. One particularly dangerous misconception: After a certain point, the damage is done and can't be erased. In reality, there are lots of simple, effective ways to minimize fine lines, erase brown spots, and firm up sagging skin.

"If you stick to just a few basics, your skin can look younger longer than you thought possible," says Dennis Gross, MD, a dermatologist in New York City and founder of the Dr. Dennis Gross Skincare line. Here, experts separate fact from fiction and reveal the best ways to keep years off your face.

Myth: Skin Should Feel Tight after Washing

TRUTH: If your skin doesn't feel fresh and supple, you're probably washing with a cleanser that's too harsh. Daily cleansing banishes blemish-causing bacteria and removes radiance robbers such as makeup, oil, and dead cells. However, harsh detergents and overwashing can increase the appearance of fine lines and can often trigger breakouts, too, as oil production kicks into overdrive to compensate for a lack of moisture. Switch to a creamy cleanser with hydrators such as glycerin as well as mild surfactants like sodium or disodium cocoyl glutamate or cocamidopropyl PG-dimonium chloride phosphate (CPG), which are derived from coconut oil.

"They all wash away makeup but restore moisture, too," says Marianna Blyumin-Karasik, MD, a clinical instructor of dermatology at the University of Miami. Try Avalon Organics Lavender Renewal Facial Cleansing Gel ($12; drugstores) and Origins Never A Dull Moment Skin-Brightening Face Cleanser ($18.50; www.origins.com).

Myth: Drugstore Products Aren't as Good

TRUTH: "Regardless of where they're sold, most antiaging lines contain the same ingredients," says David Bank, MD, a dermatologist in Mount Kisco, New York. These include scientifically proven antiagers such as retinoids, alpha hydroxy acids, peptides, and antioxidants (like vitamin C and green tea).

(continued)

To get the most bang for your buck, look for packaging designed to maintain a product's freshness and potency. For example, an airless pump keeps oxygen (and your fingers!) out of a cream, while an opaque coating around a bottle blocks sunlight. Another tip to boost effectiveness: Check the ingredient label to be sure the rejuvenators you want are listed high up—ideally, within the top 10.

Myth: Antiagers Make Skin Look Worse

TRUTH: Topical creams won't leave skin as red and blotchy as either of the big anti-aging guns—lasers or chemical peels. But key rejuvenators like retinoids, which speed cell turnover and stimulate collagen production, can be so irritating you might just want to give up.

Don't! These simple tricks will keep you from hoisting the white flag:

First-timers should prep skin for 2 weeks with an antioxidant like green tea. Try June Jacobs Advanced Cell Repair Serum ($78; www.junejacobs.com).

Consider opting for a milder OTC retinol instead of a stronger Rx version. Try Vichy LiftActiv Retinol HA Night ($42; drugstores).

Mix a pea-size amount of retinol with your face cream to help offset dryness, and apply it every second or third night.

Skin still too dry? Build up tolerance for a few weeks by putting the cream on for 5 minutes every other night and then rinsing it off. As skin becomes acclimated, work up to full nightly applications.

Myth: After Age 40, Sunscreen Is Pointless

TRUTH: By now, your skin has seen only about half its lifetime sun exposure. So don't put away the SPF. There's still plenty of time to ward off sun-induced aging. Bonus: Protecting your skin on a daily basis allows it to repair itself from past assaults.

Surprisingly, most of the damage isn't from baking on the beach. It's the result of cumulative, incidental UV exposure from, say, a quick drive to the supermarket or a midday walk.

Besides damaging skin directly, "UV rays trigger free radicals, destructive molecules that act like little darts, poking holes in skin's support structure that lead to lines and sagging," says Dr. Gross. The protection in a daily lotion with built-in sunscreen might not be enough, though. Even when the SPF is 30 or above, these formulas often lack adequate coverage against UVA rays, the main culprit behind skin aging.

To fully safeguard your skin, wear a separate sunscreen over your face cream or choose a moisturizer with avobenzone, Mexoryl, or zinc oxide, the best UVA blockers. Two sunscreens that contain potent UVA protection and antioxidants are Neutrogena Ultra Sheer Liquid Sunblock Fluid SPF 55 ($12; drugstores) and La Roche-Posay Anthelios 45 Ultra-Light Sunscreen Fluid ($30; CVS).

Myth: If a Product Doesn't Work Quickly, Move On

TRUTH: It's crucial to stick to a regimen long enough to see what works for your skin and what doesn't.

"I suggest waiting 8 to 10 weeks before you abandon a product and try the next thing," says Mark G. Rubin, MD, an assistant professor of dermatology at the University of California, San Diego, and author of *Your Skin, Younger*. And keep in mind that not everyone's skin will respond the same way to an antiager. "Most active ingredients do work on everyone—just to varying degrees," he says.

CHAPTER 29

The Pretty Skin Diet

Best fruit, best veggie, best protein. These 10 foods don't just rejuvenate skin—they deliver important health benefits to boot

Can you really eat your way to younger-looking skin? You bet!

The foods in your kitchen are just as important for keeping skin soft, smooth, and glowing as the creams in your bathroom.

"Good nutrition is a fundamental building block of healthy skin," says Leslie Baumann, MD, a Miami Beach dermatologist. The natural ingredients in food help do everything from speed the pace of exfoliation to protect skin from the UV damage that causes brown spots and wrinkles. The recipe for complexion perfection starts with a well-rounded diet of healthy fats, sufficient protein, and lots of fruits and veggies. But it also includes a bevy of power foods that feed your skin in beautiful ways.

As a bonus, these nutritional superstars also do wonders for the rest of your body—build brainpower, lower cholesterol, improve sleep, and more.

Ready to take the inside-out approach to loving your skin for life? Say hello to your new grocery list.

TOP VEGETABLE: ROMAINE LETTUCE

Why you'll glow: Six leaves provide more than 100 percent of your Daily Value of vitamin A, which revitalizes skin by increasing cell turnover.

The mineral potassium in romaine "gives skin a refreshing boost of nutrients and oxygen by improving circulation," says Lisa Drayer, RD, author of *The Beauty Diet*.

Health bonus: That same serving of romaine contains 45 percent of the DV of vitamin K, which a recent study shows activates a protein that supports vascular health—making a future with bulging leg veins less likely.

Runner-Up: Tomatoes

Why you'll glow: Eating red helps keep skin from turning red. Volunteers who consumed 5 tablespoons of high-in-lycopene tomato paste daily for 3 months had nearly 25 percent more protection against sunburn in one study. Even better, skin had more collagen, which prevents sagging.

Another reason to toss an extra tomato into your salad: German scientists report that higher skin levels of this antioxidant correlate to fewer fine lines and furrows.

Health bonus: Research suggests that lycopene may also lower your chances of heart disease: In one study, women with the highest levels of it had a 34 percent reduced risk.

TOP FRUIT: STRAWBERRIES

Why you'll glow: A cup has up to 130 percent of the DV of vitamin C, a potent antioxidant that boosts production of collagen fibers that help keep skin smooth and firm. More C may mean fewer fine lines, too: Women with lower intakes were likelier to have dry, wrinkled skin. Early research also shows that ellagic acid, an antioxidant abundant in strawberries, protects the elastic fibers that keep skin from sagging. Sweet!

Health bonus: Strawberries may lower your risk of cancer by inhibiting the development of malignant cancer cells. In one study, people eating the most strawberries were three times less likely to develop the disease.

Runner-Up: Apples

Why you'll glow: Quercetin, an antioxidant in the peel of many varieties, provides hefty protection from the "burning" UVB rays that trigger skin cancer. A few offering the biggest dose: Monroe, Cortland, and Golden Delicious. The next time you plan to spend time in the sun, pick one of them to start your day. (Of course, you still need to wear sunscreen.)

Health bonus: Eating two or more apples a week for 1 year reduced the risk of dying from heart disease by 15 percent in one study of 34,000 healthy postmenopausal women. Whatever variety you choose, be sure to eat the peel, which is the source of nearly all the antioxidants.

TOP PROTEIN: SOY

Why you'll glow: Fine wrinkles and skin firmness improved after women in their late thirties and early forties ate foods like tempeh that contain the soy isoflavone known as aglycone, found one study. Volunteers consumed an amount of aglycone comparable to 3 ounces of tempeh a day for 12 weeks.

Health bonus: Adding soy to your diet might reduce your risk of developing endometrial and ovarian cancers and diabetes and prevent a recurrence of breast cancer, finds new research. The best sources: whole foods. Try substituting edamame for any vegetable and tempeh or tofu for meat and poultry in stir-fries and soups.

Runner-Up: Eggs

Why you'll glow: Lutein and zeaxanthin, two antioxidants found in eggs, more than quadrupled protection against the UV damage that leads to lines, brown spots, and cancer in one study on women. Skin was also markedly softer, firmer, and better hydrated.

Health bonus: Eating just one egg a day significantly increases blood levels of lutein and zeaxanthin (but not cholesterol), which may stave off macular degeneration by protecting the retina from light damage, finds a study in the *Journal of Nutrition*.

TOP NUT: ALMONDS

Why you'll glow: "Eating a handful of almonds every day boosts levels of vitamin E, one of the most important antioxidants for skin health," says Dr. Baumann. You'll get a surge in moisture, too—a boon for those prone to dryness.

Health bonus: Though nuts are high in calories, women who ate them at least twice a week were less likely to gain weight than those who rarely did, according to a new study of over 50,000 women.

Runner-Up: Walnuts

Why you'll glow: These nuts are storehouses of alpha-linolenic acid, an omega-3 fat that's a key component of the lubricating layer that keeps skin moist and supple. A ½-ounce serving of walnuts provides 100 percent of the recommended daily intake of ALA.

Health bonus: Eating walnuts at dinner may deliver better shut-eye. Researchers at the University of Texas Health Science Center discovered that walnuts contain melatonin, a hormone that regulates sleep.

TOP FAT: COCOA MADE WITH DARK CHOCOLATE

Why you'll glow: Women in one study positively glowed after drinking ½ cup, thanks to a significant increase in circulation that lasted 2 hours. But a daily cocoa habit might rejuvenate your complexion even more. Women who drank ½ cup of cocoa high in flavonoids (as is dark chocolate) every day for 12 weeks in another study had significantly softer, smoother, and better hydrated skin. Try Nestlé Hot Cocoa Dark Chocolate.

Health bonus: An 8-ounce cup of cocoa improved bloodflow to the brain for 2 hours in British research. Besides better functioning on complex tasks, participants showed more brain activity in MRI scans, which is an indication of enhanced brain function that might reduce the risk of dementia.

Runner-Up: Extra-Virgin Olive Oil

Why you'll glow: This healthy fat contains essential fatty acids that help skin resist UV damage, finds a *Lancet Oncology* study. EFAs are also part of the cell membranes that help hold in moisture. The body can't synthesize EFAs, so consume about 1 tablespoon of olive oil daily to keep skin supple.

Health bonus: Recent research suggests that hydroxytyrosol, a component in olive oil, lowers cholesterol and helps prevent obesity and diabetes by revving the energy centers in your cells. Using it in meals also warded off the next round of hunger pains in one study, so you're less likely to snack.

CHAPTER 30

Every Day Is a Good Skin Day

Here's how the best skin experts look their best—and how you can, too

Tempted to corner the dermatologist you meet at a cocktail party for her best skin-saving advice? No need. We asked top experts in the field how they keep their skin young, fresh, and glowing 24/7.

Look sun-kissed. "A little tint takes years off your face by evening out your skin tone," which a recent study found is a key marker of youthfulness, says Ranella Hirsch, MD, a dermatologist in Cambridge, Massachusetts.

Her favorite for a natural look: Olay Complete Touch of Sun Daily UV Moisturizer + A Touch of Sunless Tanner ($15; drugstores), a lotion with a low level of self-tanner.

Eat a skin-saving breakfast. The first meal of the day for New York City derm Doris Day, MD, includes almonds.

"They contain essential fatty acids, which help put the brakes on inflammation that accelerates fine lines, sagging, and blotchiness." Not feeling like a nut? Salmon, tuna, and halibut are good lunch and dinner sources.

Spray away dryness. To keep her skin supple, Los Angeles–based derm Jessica Wu, MD, sprays it several times daily with La Roche-Posay Thermal Spring Water ($9; drugstores). (She often spritzes her face when stuck in traffic!)

Bonus: The water is packed with minerals such as selenium that protect against UV damage.

Pour on the protection. To ensure she layers on enough sunscreen ("the best way to keep skin youthful"), Garland, Texas–based dermatologist Lisa Garner, MD, president of the Women's Dermatologic Society, fills the hollow of her palm (about ½ teaspoon) with a broad-spectrum sunscreen with SPF 30 or higher to coat her face, neck, and ears.

"I usually have to apply two coats to finish what I've squeezed out, but that's how I make sure I'm covered."

Zen your skin. If anyone has stress, it's doctors. High levels of tension can spike hormone production that leads to breakouts or aggravates conditions such as psoriasis.

"Controlling stress keeps your skin calm, but that's easier said than done," says Annie Chiu, MD, a derm in Los Angeles. Taking a 10-minute time-out to apply a face mask and relax on her bed works for Chiu. Another trick: Ban the 'Berry. "I turn off my cell phone after 8:00 at night. Every little bit helps!" she says.

Protect with powder. Sunscreen stops working in less than 3 hours, so reapplication is key, says Washington, DC–based derm Elizabeth Tanzi, MD. For easy touch-ups, she uses powder sunscreen.

"It's light, so makeup stays intact." Her fave: Colorescience Pro Sunforgettable Powder SPF 50 ($60; www.colorescience.com).

Develop a bedside manner. "I often find it difficult to stick to my antiaging regimen at bedtime," says Francesca Fusco, MD, a New York City derm. To avoid missing her evening routine, she stores these products in a pretty makeup case she keeps on her nightstand. "So if I've forgotten—or was just too tired to apply products at the sink—I can do it easily while in bed." Her must-haves: Renova (a prescription retinoid), EpiCeram (an ultrahydrating Rx moisturizer), SCO lip balm, Earth to Skin Care Cracked Heel Renewal, Creative Nail Design SolarOil (to soften cuticles), and Listerine Whitening Strips.

Wear your veggies. Frozen peas help soothe itchy, irritated eyes for Jeanine Downie, MD, a derm in Montclair, New Jersey. "Once I get home from work, I remove my makeup and put a bag of frozen peas on my lids for about 5 minutes."

The cold helps reduce swelling and pigmentation, which is a side effect of repeated irritation from her eczema. Unlike inflexible ice packs, a bag of peas easily conforms to the shape of the eyes for a faster effect.

Avoid impact. "The repeated jarring of high-impact cardio like running can weaken collagen and lead to sagging," says Oakland, California, dermatologist Katie Rodan, MD. "So until a 'face bra' is invented, I'll stick to cycling and the elliptical machine."

Strike a pose. Most derms will bend over backward for great skin. Hema Sundaram, MD, a Washington, DC–area dermatologist, bends forward. Yoga moves like Child's Pose, Downward-Facing Dog, and Sun Salutations improve circulation—the boost of oxygen is what gives skin that lovely "yoga glow."

Another reason to take to the mat: New research finds regular yoga practice may reduce the inflammation and stress that speed skin aging.

Lather with care. "Mild cleansers are one of my best secrets," says Chicago derm Jonith Breadon, MD. She's partial to CeraVe Hydrating Cleanser ($12; drugstores), which contains ceramides—fatty materials that help retain moisture.

Cut back on the sweet stuff. The breakdown of sugars, called glycation, damages the collagen that keeps skin smooth and firm. To prevent this natural process from careening out of control, Naila Malik, MD, a derm in Southlake, Texas, sticks to low-glycemic carbs such as whole grains. They're naturally low in sugar, and the body processes them slowly, limiting the loss of collagen.

Pump iron to plump skin. "I am religious about strength training, and I always tell patients to do it more as they get older," says Patricia Farris, MD, a dermatologist in Metairie, Louisiana. The payoff: firmer skin from the neck down, the result of having better, more supportive muscle tone.

"It's like adding volume to the face with fillers, except on your body," says Dr. Farris.

CHAPTER 31

Flower Power

The following botanical beauties put the bloom back into aging skin

These days, skin care is coming up roses—and daffodils, cornflowers, and echinacea. That's because their petals, stems, bulbs, and oils are the cures for myriad complexion concerns. Here are some potent potions to try.

FEVERFEW: REDUCES REDNESS

Named for its traditional use as a fever reducer, this daisylike flower is a proven anti-inflammatory and antioxidant, ideal for soothing sensitive skin and reducing redness—both of which become more common after age 35. Studies on people with sensitive skin found significant improvement in redness, irritation, and roughness after they applied a product with feverfew twice daily.

It's so good at calming skin that Jessica Wu, MD, an assistant clinical professor of dermatology at the University of Southern California Medical School, has patients with sensitive skin use it to minimize the dryness and scaliness caused by age-erasing retinoids.

Try Philosophy Amazing Grace Perfumed Body Spritz ($25; www.philosophy.com), Neutrogena Ageless Restoratives Anti-Oxidant Daily Moisturizer SPF 20 ($19; www.neutrogena.com), the Aveeno Ultra-Calming skin care line (from $8; drugstores), and First Aid Beauty Ultra Repair Cream ($28; www.firstaidbeauty.com).

ECHINACEA: CLEARS ACNE

Best known as a natural cold fighter, echinacea was used by Native Americans and early settlers to treat skin infections, wounds, and stings. Today, science backs up these benefits: One study of 4,500 people with inflammatory skin conditions (including psoriasis) reported an 85 percent cure rate with topical application of echinacea.

This colorful herb is commonly used to allay acne by killing bacteria and reducing swelling. It's particularly helpful for grownups battling breakouts and wrinkles: Echinacea is rich in echinacein, a substance that assists fibroblasts (the cells that create skin-smoothing collagen) in working more efficiently.

Try Korres Echinacea Soap for Oily Skin ($8.50; www.korresusa.com), Noah's Naturals Pore Refining Masque ($9; Walmart), and Terressentials Organic Flower Therapy Exfoliating Facial Toner ($17; www.terressentials.com).

EVENING PRIMROSE: EASES ECZEMA AND PSORIASIS

The lightweight oil extracted from the seeds of this wildflower quells the itching, dryness, and scaliness of eczema and psoriasis, show a number of studies. Its soothing nature comes from a rich supply of linoleic acid and gamma linoleic acid, essential fatty acids that are key players in keeping skin hydrated.

Their other important role: to assist in the production of prostaglandins, substances that regulate inflammation. Because psoriasis and eczema sufferers tend to have abnormally low levels of gamma linoleic acid, any boost can be helpful.

Try Kiehl's Midnight Recovery Concentrate ($43; www.kiehls.com), Aubrey Organics Evening Primrose Soothing Moisturizing Lotion ($14; www.aubrey-organics.com), and Tree Hut Shea Sugar Body Scrub ($7; www.drugstore.com).

CORNFLOWER: SOOTHES PUFFY EYES

This brilliant blue flower boasts a long history as the go-to remedy for eye troubles. Even today, practitioners of herbal medicine treat conjunctivitis with a cornflower eyewash and relieve strain by applying a poultice of petals over the eyes. Studies explain why it's a natural for peeper problems: Besides being antibacterial, the flower heads contain several anti-inflammatory substances, says a *Journal of Ethnopharmacology* study.

Try Vichy Laboratoires Purete Thermale Eye Make-Up Remover for Sensitive Eyes ($15; drugstores), Klorane Cornflower Smoothing and Relaxing Patches ($18; www.beauty.com), and Talika Eye Dream Regenerator Night Mask ($55; www.talika.com).

DAFFODIL: DEFEATS DRYNESS

An extract of the daffodil bulb called IBR-Dormin ends the cycle of dryness by normalizing the rate at which cells are produced. When skin is dry, cells form too fast to be healthy.

"This extract helps the daffodil bulb go dormant by slowing the creation of cells; when it wears off, cell production begins," explains Helen Knaggs, PhD, vice president of global research and development at Nu Skin. The extract has a similar effect on skin: "Cells need enough time to develop so they're able to hold in moisture."

Try Elizabeth Arden Intervene Radiance Boosting Moisture Cream SPF 15 ($49; www.shop.elizabetharden.com) and Tata Harper Restorative Eye Crème ($90; www.tataharperskincare.com).

CHAPTER 32

Natural Hair Makeovers

Trim away the years! These miracle hair makeovers are cheaper and faster than a face-lift!

Is it any wonder that most women say that on a "good hair day" they feel great? On a "bad hair day," not so much. If you can find the right cut and color, you'll look 10 years younger in 30 minutes flat.

According to a survey conducted by Clairol, almost half of women— 47 percent—report that their hair determines whether or not they feel beautiful. We completely understand!

"I FEEL PEPPIER. IT'S LIKE A NEW BEGINNING."

Sandy Schocker, 52, operating room nurse, Hollidaysburg, Pennsylvania

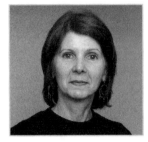

Then: The volume in Sandy's style was centered at her jaw, highlighting an area prone to sagging. Melissa Bridgers, color director at New York City's OC61 Salon, thought a richer hair hue would be more flattering.

Wow! Cutting graduated layers and feathery bangs redirects attention up toward Sandy's pretty eyes. "The effect is soft and youthful," says OC61 artistic director Louise O'Connor. A warm copper hair color allows Sandy's bright eyes and beautiful skin to shine through.

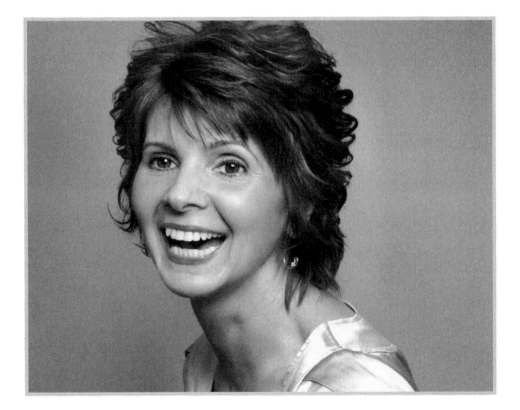

5-Second Makeup Age Erasers

On her cheeks: "Switch to a cream blush for a moist glow," says makeup artist Lynn LaMorte. To keep blush from fading, moisturize before applying, and brush on translucent loose powder to set. Try Mac Blushcreme in Posey ($18.50; maccosmetics.com).

On her lips: Sandy's vibrant hair color calls for a lipstick in a similar tone, such as berry. "Anything too pink can look garish with red hair," says LaMorte. Tip: To achieve a pretty, "stained" effect, tap on lipstick with your finger rather than swiping.

Try This at Home

First, O'Connor spritzed Sandy's hair with a thickening spray. Try Phytovolume Actif Volumizing Spray ($28; www.sephora.com).

She used a small round brush to blow-dry Sandy's hair up and off her face. Try Umberto's Round Brush #103 ($11; Target).

To keep Sandy's 'do from looking too "set," O'Connor used a curling iron "here and there" for a tousled texture. Try Infiniti by Conair You Curl Tourmaline Ceramic Curling Iron ($50; drugstores).

33 THE PERCENTAGE OF WOMEN WHO STICK TO ONE SHAMPOO BRAND

"MY HAIR LOOKS HEALTHIER AND FEELS SO SILKY!"

Eliana Delucia, 57, sales associate, Hewitt, New Jersey

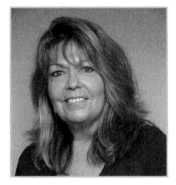

Then: Eliana's hair had little movement, which is an instant ager, because a stiff 'do looks old-fashioned. Plus, her wispy bangs were out of proportion to the rest of her hair. And a lack of contrast between her base shade and highlights resulted in a drab effect.

FACE-SLIMMING STYLES

There's no such thing as instant weight loss, but the right haircut comes close. Ask your stylist about these tricks from Harry Josh, stylist and international creative consultant for John Frieda.

- Side parts and side-swept bangs make fuller faces look less round.
- Adding volume at the crown slims by drawing the eye upward.
- Angled face-framing layers cut an inch below your jawline define cheekbones and camouflage a double chin.
- Straight locks elongate your physique.

Wow! Snipping Eliana's hair to her shoulders and adding face-framing pieces makes her look closer to 50 than 60.

"The length adds softness around her chin and neck [bonus: layers help camouflage this area], and the fringe hides forehead furrows," says O'Connor. To make Eliana's color pop, Bridgers deepened her base, added blonde highlights, and finished with a sheer gold gloss that makes her skin glow.

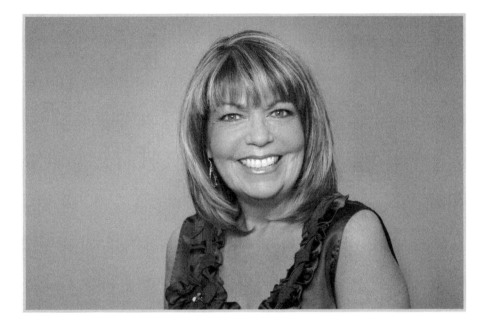

5-Second Makeup Age Eraser

To visually lift hooded eyelids, apply a medium brown matte eye shadow to the area just above the crease. Stroke a shimmery champagne shade on the brow bone to highlight it.

Try This at Home

O'Connor applied a styling cream for shine and smoothness. Try Living Proof No Frizz Styling Cream ($24; www.sephora.com).

She used a volumizing spray and blow-dried the roots to lock in the lift. Try Garnier Fructis Style Body Boost Root Booster ($4; drugstores).

"MY TEENAGE SON SAID NOW I LOOK LIKE I'M 30!"

Desta Lakew, 46, fundraiser, Ossining, New York

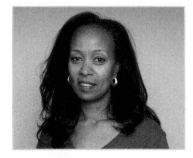

Then: "A one-length hairstyle is the hardest to wear as you get older. It can age you by a decade," says O'Connor. "Adding bangs and layers instantly updates the look." Desta's dark, monochromatic hair color can also look harsh against aging skin, says colorist Tiffanie Richards.

COOL SECRET FOR HEALTHY HAIR

Your curling iron and straightener may have a dirty little secret: Product buildup can burn hair and cause split ends, according to Aussie celebrity stylist Sarah Potempa. Clean tools weekly this way:

First, turn them on for a second; the warmth makes the film easier to wipe away. Turn them back off! Then dip a cloth in rubbing alcohol and run it over the metal plates. This removes any residue but keeps the protective coating intact, so hair won't fry. Dry immediately with a fresh cloth to prevent rusting.

60 THE PERCENTAGE OF WOMEN WHO USE HEATED TOOLS LIKE A FLATIRON AT LEAST ONCE A WEEK, ACCORDING TO DOVE

Wow! O'Connor snipped off about 8 inches and added graduated layers to frame Desta's face. "Wearing hair above the shoulder is much sexier," says O'Connor. Because Desta has a high forehead, O'Connor went with side-swept bangs for a softer overall effect. Richards wove caramel highlights through Desta's hair, so it looks "like a light is shining on it."

5-Second Makeup Age Eraser

To cover dark spots, dab on concealer after applying foundation so you won't rub it off while blending in foundation, says LaMorte. Choose a shade slightly lighter than your skin. Try Make Up For Ever Full Cover Concealer ($30; www.sephora.com).

Try This at Home

O'Connor worked a styling cream into Desta's wet hair. Try Moroccanoil Hydrating Styling Cream ($32; see www.moroccanoil.com for salon locations).

She used a round brush while blow-drying, then went over with a flatiron. Try Cricket Friction Free Flat Iron ($43; www.sallybeauty.com).

"THIS NEW CUT IS DEFINITELY THE CONFIDENCE BOOSTER I NEEDED"

Nancy Bogdan, 53, accountant, Queens, New York

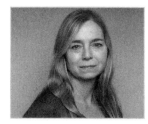

Then: "I've worn my hair this way since junior high school," wrote Nancy, who wanted a more sophisticated style as she embarked on a new career as a self-employed small business owner. Though her long locks were easy to care for (Nancy even trimmed them herself!), "her hair just hung there and didn't do anything to play up her beautiful eyes and bone structure," says O'Connor.

Wow! Chopping off 6 inches—Nancy's limit—gave her an instant lift. Bonus: Going shorter made her fine hair look thicker—a big plus because hair becomes even finer with age, making the ends seem straggly. Bangs brought the focus to her stunning eyes. Nancy's naturally blonde hair had grown darker but not very gray with age. Richards wove in chunky blonde highlights to add brightness and the illusion of more depth—another boost for limp hair. "It looks natural but polished," says Richards.

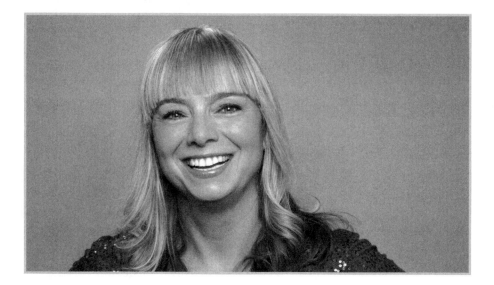

5-Second Makeup Age Erasers

On her eyes: LaMorte used a complementary peachy shadow to bring out Nancy's vibrant blue eyes. Got green eyes? Try plum, aubergine, or grayish purples. For brown eyes, go for golds, bronzes, and olives. To bring out a fleck of gold in any eye color, opt for navy liner.

On her lips: Skip the frosted lipstick and opt for a creamy formula. "Frosted textures accentuate skin flaws," explains LaMorte. Try Rimmel London Moisture Renew Lip Colour in Rose Blush ($7; drugstores).

Try This at Home

O'Connor spritzed Nancy's locks with a volumizing spray to give her hair some heft. Try Pantene Pro-V Fine Hair Style Root Lifter Spray Gel ($4; drugstores).

She blow-dried Nancy's hair using a brush with a ceramic-coated barrel. Try Marilyn Jeli Ceramica Brush ($24 to $38; www.marilynbrush.com).

If fine hair looks oily, spray on a dry shampoo. "It will give your blowout another day or two of staying power," says O'Connor. Try Suave Professionals Dry Shampoo ($3; drugstores).

SHAMPOO MYTH COMES CLEAN

Is it true that the same shampoo stops working well after a while?

If your mane starts misbehaving, don't fall for the shampoo-resistance rumor. "Hair is dead and can't biologically adapt to shampoo," says Jeni Thomas, PhD, a senior scientist at Pantene. But even though your hair can't get "used to" your favorite shampoo, there are reasons to switch:

- You have buildup from heavy conditioners (use a clarifying shampoo occasionally).
- You started coloring or straightening (opt for moisturizing formulas).
- The weather changed (ask your stylist for a seasonal routine).

CHAPTER 33

Beauty Sleep

Yes, you can sleep like a baby! (And wake up looking younger.) Your skin is hard at work repairing itself while you rest. Take advantage of this natural healing process with the right routine

Nighttime is the right time to take years off your face. "Hormonal changes boost bloodflow to the skin, brightening it overnight," says Melvin Elson, MD, a clinical professor of dermatology at Vanderbilt School of Nursing. Skin temps are higher, too, so age-fighting potions seep deeper for better results. And even though you're resting, your skin is hard at work. Studies show that cell turnover is eight times faster at night, softening wrinkles.

On the flip side, as anyone who's pulled an all-nighter can attest, the consequences—pasty-looking skin and dark circles—aren't pretty.

"Even worse, not getting the recommended 8 hours increases levels of the stress hormone cortisol, which may slow collagen production, promoting wrinkles," says Jyotsna Sahni, MD, a sleep medicine doctor at Canyon Ranch in Tucson.

To maximize your beauty sleep, follow this routine nightly and wake up with the complexion of your dreams.

WASH YOUR FACE

Removing makeup, oil, and other impurities helps keep pores tight and skin blemish free. Antiaging treatments can also penetrate deeper on a clean surface. For dry skin, look for a creamy cleanser; for acne-prone or oily skin, a gel formula. If your skin is sensitive, wait 10 minutes after cleansing before applying antiagers.

REJUVENATE WITH A RETINOID

These vitamin A derivatives are key to youthful-looking skin.

"But because exposure to sunlight can deactivate their potency, it's best to apply retinoids at night," says Patricia Farris, MD, an assistant clinical professor of dermatology at Tulane University School of Medicine. Start by using an OTC retinol-containing cream or lotion every other night until skin becomes acclimated to the side effects.

Try: Neutrogena Tone Correcting Concentrated Serum Night from Ageless Intensives ($22; drugstores) or La Roche-Posay Biomedic Retinol Cream 15 ($52; drugstores). For more improvement, try prescription Renova, Atralin, or Refissa, a newly available retinoid in a moisturizing base.

DOT UNDEREYES WITH VITAMIN K CREAM

In a 2003 study by Dr. Elson, women who applied an undereye cream containing vitamin K and retinol every night for 12 weeks saw their dark circles improve 33 percent.

Try: NeoStrata Bionic Eye Cream ($50; www.skinstore.com) or Murad Essential-C Eye Cream SPF 15 ($67; www.sephora.com). Like retinol, vitamin K is sensitive to ultraviolet light and should be used only at night.

Bonus: The retinol helps ease crow's-feet.

APPLY A MEGA-MOISTURIZER

Due to nighttime increase in temperature and water loss, extra hydration is a must, says Jenny Kim, MD, PhD, an associate professor of medicine and dermatology at the UCLA Department of Medicine. For best results, look for a cream with the superhydrators hyaluronic acid or glycerin, which attract water to skin. The extra dose of softening also makes wrinkles less noticeable in the morning.

Try: Mario Badescu Hydrating Moisturizer with Biocare & Hyaluronic Acid ($20; www.mariobadescu.com) or Dr. Dennis Gross Skincare Maximum Moisture Treatment ($54; www.dgskincare.com).

SOLVE YOUR SKIN PROBLEMS OVERNIGHT

You know that saying "You snooze, you lose"? Well, nothing is further from the truth when it comes to skin care. In fact, nighttime is the right time to repair aging skin and keep it ultramoisturized. "During the day, skin is in protection mode—it's busy fending off environmental aggressors like sun, wind, and pollution," says Jeannette Graf, MD, a dermatologist in Great Neck, New York. At night, while you rest, your skin has time to replenish. "This is when it does the bulk of its repair work," such as creating new cells and mending or shedding old, damaged ones, says Dr. Graf.

Your skin makes the most of any creams you apply at night, too: Because it gets warmer then, products penetrate more deeply, yielding faster results, explains David Bank, MD, a dermatologist in Mount Kisco, New York. This is a huge plus in the winter, when skin loses more than 25 percent of its ability to hold in moisture. That drop means a slowdown in skin turnover that leaves your complexion looking dull. For 40-plus women, who often already have dry skin, that can really ratchet up the problem—especially if you're also using ingredients that can irritate skin, like retinoids to control acne and aging. But don't give up on having a soft, smooth, fresh-faced glow. Our guide to choosing the right night cream goes beyond restoring lost moisture; these p.m. perfecters also contain potent antiagers that rejuvenate skin. Just pinpoint your main complexion concern and preferred texture—balm, cream, lotion, gel, or serum—and prepare to get the skin of your dreams.

YOU WANT INTENSIVE CARE FOR DRY SKIN

If your skin is tight, rough, and flaky, it's time to sub a mega-moisturizer for your regular nighttime product. Key ingredients for dehydrated skin include fatty acids, such as linolenic or linoleic acid, and ceramides to repair skin's natural moisture barrier; hyaluronic acid and glycerin to attract water to the skin; and petrolatum, mineral oil, and dimethicone to seal it in. Stick with balms or creams; most lotions aren't hydrating enough for dry skin. And remember, regular use is a must. "Moisturizers can control dry skin, not cure it," points out Mary Lupo, MD, a dermatologist in New Orleans.

20 THE PERCENTAGE OF PEOPLE WHO SLEEP FEWER THAN 6 HOURS A NIGHT

FOUR SLEEP TRICKS FOR AMAZING SKIN

Make the most of your shut-eye with these simple solutions.

SLEEP ON YOUR BACK. Lying on your stomach or on the same side every night can etch permanent sleep lines into your skin, says Patricia Farris, MD. If you can't adjust, switch to a satin pillowcase; the silky texture prevents crinkles.

RAISE YOUR HEAD. Stack a few pillows beneath your head to avoid puffy eyes. "If you keep your head above your heart, fluid won't accumulate in your face," says Dr. Farris.

INVEST IN A HUMIDIFIER. Dry, hot air sucks moisture from skin. A humidifier puts water in the air, for soft and supple skin.

GET DEEPER SLEEP. Use the bedroom for sleep and sex only. Doing so trains your mind to associate your bed with getting z's. Avoid caffeine and exercise for 3 to 5 hours before bedtime, and limit alcohol at night; each can keep you from solid slumber. Make sure your room is dark and cool (the ideal temp for sleep is 65°F). To transition into sleep mode, don't watch TV or go online for an hour before turning in.

Balms away: Collective Wellbeing Night Balm ($27; www.collectivewellbeing.com) contains echinacea to stimulate production of skin-smoothing collagen, plus lavender to help lull you into dreamland. La Roche-Posay Substiane Daily Replenishing Care for Mature Skin ($55; www.laroche-posay.us) features Pro-xylane, a sugar molecule that firms and hydrates skin.

Creams of the crop: The rose hip oil in SkinCeuticals Emollience ($59; www.skinceuticals.com) is a gentle, natural source of antiaging retinoic acid. Boots No7 Lifting & Firming Night Cream ($20; Target) contains peptides to smooth skin and prevent sagging.

Super serums: Unlike heavier creams and balms, serums can be used during the day, under your SPF and foundation. For an instant surge of moisture, try Vichy Laboratoires Aqualia Thermal Serum 24Hr Hydrating Concentrate ($31.50; www.vichyusa.com) and Philosophy When Hope Is Not Enough Replenishing Oil ($45; www.philosophy.com).

YOU WANT LESS SENSITIVE SKIN

If you suffer from rosacea, a condition that makes your skin prone to flushing and blushing, or if your skin just normally stings and burns when you apply products, you need a night cream that coddles your complexion. Fragrance aggravates sensitivity, so look for fragrance-free products, which means no scent has been added. Don't be surprised, however, if a fragrance-free product has an aroma. They often contain natural soothers such as lavender oil and rose oil. Also essential: ingredients proven to ease irritation. Some MVPs include coffeeberry, green tea, and vitamin C, antioxidants that help lessen lines and fade brown patches.

WEATHER WINTER BEAUTIFULLY

Winter can be especially hard on skin. The right night cream goes a long way to combat dryness. But to keep seasonal ravages at bay, incorporate these easy pro tips into your routine as well.

Use a humidifier in your bedroom at night. "You'll hydrate your skin continuously while you sleep," says Ranella Hirsch, MD.

Exfoliate extra gently. "Removing flaky, dead cells helps moisturizers penetrate better," says Mary Lupo, MD. Daily exfoliation is ideal. Try Philosophy Microdelivery Exfoliating Wash ($25; www.sephora.com), which is mild enough for even the most sensitive skin.

Wash your face only at night, using a nonfoaming cleanser. In the morning, splash your skin with tepid water or apply your moisturizer first and then rinse it off, suggests Dr. Lupo.

Moisturize immediately after cleansing, while skin is still damp, to help trap water in the surface cells.

Eat more salmon. "The omega-3 fatty acids in fish are skin's natural emollient," says Dr. Hirsch. Other good sources of omega-3s: walnuts, canola oil, and ground flaxseed.

WAKE UP LOOKING YOUNGER!

Studies show that sleeping on a pillow in the same position night after night creates wrinkles that can take hours to go away—or even become permanent. To the rescue: the Mumbani Fresh Face ($25; www.mumbani.com), a cushioned pillow you wear like a sleep mask to minimize pressure on your face. Our tester woke up with fewer crinkles and claims to have slept better, too. Independent research confirms her experience—75 percent of users saw smoother skin, and more than half reported sounder slumber.

Balms away: Eau Thermale Avène Tolerance Extreme Cream ($36; www.dermstore.com) has an airtight cap that eliminates the need for preservatives, another potential skin aggravator. Vichy Laboratoires Aqualia Thermal Mineral Balm ($34; www.vichyusa.com) contains water rich in selenium, a mineral proven to reduce inflammation.

Creams of the crop: Aveeno Positively Ageless Night Cream with Active Naturals Natural Shiitake Complex ($20; drugstores) features mushroom extracts that slough dead cells to enhance luminosity. Boscia Restorative Night Moisture Cream ($48; www.sephora.com) is loaded with botanical extracts—willow herb, rose, and mulberry—to quell inflammation and brighten skin.

Lotions you'll love: CeraVe Facial Moisturizing Lotion PM ($13; drugstores) is packed with niacinamide, a B vitamin that reduces redness and minimizes dark spots. Dr. Lupo also recommends using coffeeberry, found in Priori CoffeeBerry Night Complex ($84; www.prioriskincare.com for buying info), during the day under SPF to squelch UV-induced free radicals.

Super serums: Those with vitamin C—like Murad Sensitive Skin Soothing Serum ($49.50; www.murad.com) and Paula's Choice Resist Super Antioxidant Concentrate Serum ($25; www.paulaschoice.com)—ramp up collagen production and tone down discoloration.

YOU WANT A MOISTURIZER THAT DOESN'T MAKE YOU BREAK OUT

It's easy to think you don't need a rich night cream when you're battling blemishes. But after age 40, everyone needs extra hydration in the winter—especially if you're also using drying acne treatments. Your mission: Choose a product that quenches skin without causing pimples. It's not enough to opt for noncomedogenic products, which means they won't block pores, says Dr. Bank.

"Scan the ingredients carefully for oil in any form—even some natural oils like safflower oil can trigger breakouts." Hydrators to look for include hyaluronic acid, glycerin, and dimethicone; even alpha hydroxy acids such as lactic and glycolic acids, which exfoliate dead cells to clear pores, are mildly moisturizing. Skip heavy balms, which usually contain oil. A new category of moisturizer is ideal if you're blemish-prone: hydragels, which have a lightweight gel base.

Creams of the crop: Kate Somerville Oil Free Moisturizer ($65; www.katesomerville.com) contains an algae extract that firms skin while you sleep. Pürminerals Moisture Infusion ($34; www.drugstore.com) minimizes the inflammation of *P. acnes* bacteria with green tea.

Lotions you'll love: Dr. Brandt Blemishes No More Oil-Free Hydrator ($35; www.sephora.com) contains peptides to firm, hydroxycinnamic acid to even tone, and salicylic acid to clear pores and make you look glowy. If you're acne-prone and sensitive, DDF Ultra Lite Oil Free Moisturizing Dew ($38; www.sephora.com) provides relief with calming ingredients like aloe and allantoin.

Swell gels: To minimize pores, Avon Anew Rejuvenate Night Sapphire Emulsion ($30; www.shop.avon.com) taps the power of peptides and salicylic acid. The vitamin E in Garnier Nutritioniste Moisture Rescue Refreshing Gel-Cream ($8; drugstores) soothes and protects against free radicals.

Super serums: When skin is parched from acne meds, Epicuren Moisture Surge Hyaluronic Acid Gel ($28; see www.epicuren.com for store locations) and Peter Thomas Roth VIZ-1000 ($65; www.sephora.com) flood it with hyaluronic acid—which acts like a magnet to bind water to skin.

FIVE WAYS TO LOOK BRIGHT-EYED

Battle every cause of dark circles—aging, allergies, and exhaustion—with the following pro tips.

WHITE EYE PENCIL: Apply to inner eye corners to instantly brighten a dark area women often miss, says London-based makeup artist Liz Pugh. Focus around tear ducts and the hollows of your nose, smudging with your pinky to soften the effect. Try Rimmel Soft Kohl Kajal Eye Liner Pencil in Pure White ($4, drugstores).

EYE CREAM: Dark circles may appear when thin skin reveals veins underneath. Look for a cream with peptides to build collagen and caffeine to constrict blood vessels. Try GoodSkin Labs Eyliplex-2 Eye Lift + Circle Reducer ($40, www.kohls.com).

CONCEALER: Choose a yellow-toned cover-up one or two shades lighter than your skin. Apply with a small brush only to dark areas—if you also lighten surrounding skin, circles still look darker by comparison. Try L'Oreal Paris Visible Lift Line-Minimizing & Tone-Enhancing Concealer with SPF 20 ($12, drugstores).

ALLERGY FIX: Try an antihistamine and a decongestant to fade allergy-induced darkness within a month. A med-free solution: Sleep with two pillows to keep blood from pooling under eyes.

A DISTRACTION: To take the focus off circles, don't line or apply mascara to lower lashes. Instead, redirect attention with a brighter blush or lipstick.

YOU WANT AN ANTIAGING BOOST

If your night cream is marvelous at moisturizing but isn't up to the job of fading brown splotches and reducing lines and wrinkles, you don't need to switch creams. Instead, pat on an antiaging serum prior to moisturizing.

"Topping a serum with a cream or lotion actually seals in its active ingredients—and reduces the chance they'll rub off on your pillow," says Ranella Hirsch, MD, a dermatologist in Cambridge, Massachusetts. Keep in mind that winter isn't the season to start using a retinoid, which can be an especially drying antiager. Better ingredients to look for: peptides, which boost collagen production to plump skin; lactic acid and glycolic acid to speed cell renewal and rev radiance; and brighteners like licorice and vitamin C to fade brown spots.

Super serums: MD Formulations Continuous Renewal Serum ($53; www.bareescentuals.com) gently polishes skin with glycolic acid. Got sensitive skin? Olay Regenerist Fragrance-Free Regenerating Serum ($20; drugstores), with niacinamide and peptides, is ideal. To stop early signs of aging, Clinique Repairwear Laser Focus Wrinkle & UV Damage Corrector ($44.50; www.clinique.com) calls on peptides, antioxidants, and repair enzymes.

journal

HEALTHY RULES TO LIVE BY

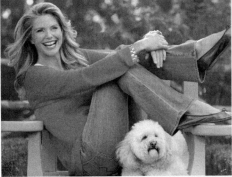

Who wouldn't want to look as great and glowing as Christie Brinkley does—at 56, no less? Expensive creams and fitness trainers are not her secrets. Instead, it's these 10 humble and wholesome insights.

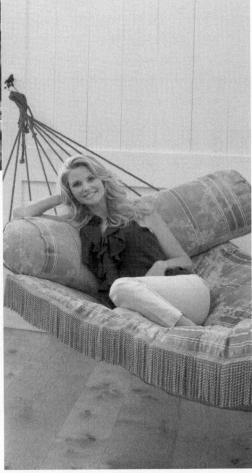

Long before androgynous-looking waifs or silicone-enhanced supermodels strutted the runways, there was Christie Brinkley. Genetically blessed with high cheekbones, big blue eyes, thick blonde hair, a dazzling smile, and a sculpted body, the sunny California girl epitomized easy, natural beauty.

But beyond the glossy high-def image, Brinkley has also made a name for herself as an enthusiastic and vocal supporter of environmental causes, from eating local and organic to preserving our oceans. In addition to raising three children and caring for her ailing parents, she's had more than her share of challenges: four marriages (the last one ending in the glare of publicity surrounding her divorce from philandering architect Peter Cook), a helicopter crash in the 1990s, major back surgery. It's a lot for anyone to live through.

Yet through all her travails, Brinkley has retained not only her genuine smile but the kind of optimism that leads to, as she puts it, "being overwhelmed by the miracle of a flower" when she steps out of her house in the morning. What on Earth is she putting into the lemonade she keeps making from life's lemons? For the recipe, we went straight to the source: Here are Christie Brinkley's personal rules for staying not only sane but also happy and healthy.

Everything Is about Family

Part of what keeps her grounded, Brinkley says, is the clear understanding that her children (Alexa Ray, 25; Jack, 15; and Sailor, 12) take precedence. "I always knew I wanted to be a mother," Brinkley says. Make no mistake, she adds, "it takes a lot of work." And sometimes it's being away from her family that makes her appreciate being around them all the more. "My work makes me a better mom. It gives me a little door to step out of my parenting and bring the excitement from that day back home." For Brinkley, it's not just about her kids, either. Her parents have relocated from California to New York so Brinkley can keep an eye on them, too. (Her father suffers from Parkinson's disease, while her mother has survived a series of strokes.) "Despite the challenges, they're incredibly strong," says Brinkley. Her experience with her parents' illnesses has informed Brinkley's support of stem cell research. "I would love for it to get the funding that's needed," she says.

You Gotta Have Friends

Then there is that other family: the one that's made up of your most trusted confidantes. "When you have great friendships, talking out a problem just isn't a big deal," says Brinkley, "because you know in your heart you'd do the same for them."

Brinkley should know. When she divorced Cook, it was her pals who helped her navigate some rough seas. "You've got to find a way to keep laughing, even if it's black humor, and my friends are very good at that." And don't discount the pure fun factor: "Some people think of happiness as a luxury, but it's a necessity, and you need to make space for it in your life." So is she making space for another romantic relationship? It's complicated, says Brinkley. "Most of the time, I've got my kids with me, so I'm not as prone to meeting people. And then, you never really know if someone is talking to you because you're a celebrity. It's not my number one priority."

Get Into "Move Groove"

When you consider Brinkley's she-can't-really-be-56 figure, you know physical activity has to come into it somewhere. But it's not just about her shape, she insists; it's about how she feels. "It's when I'm inactive that I notice the aches and pains that creep in with my age," says Brinkley. So she moves on all fronts: quick workouts on her Total Gym (equipment that "simulates yoga and Pilates moves") and tennis, yoga, skiing. "I like to mix it up so I don't get bored." And she steals whatever moments she can. "When I'm walking on the beach, I'll sneak in some lunges or squats as I bend down to pick up shells. I don't care if it looks silly!"

Never Say "Diet"

Brinkley's approach to eating is similarly holistic. There are no extreme remedies here (being a nearly lifelong vegetarian is as fringe as it gets), just a series of small decisions throughout the day that balance pleasure and moderation. "Saying you're on a diet puts you in the frame of denying yourself," she explains. "But if you replace 'diet' with 'healthy choices,' you're giving yourself the gift of feeling good." And sometimes the healthiest choice is a piece of chocolate. "Go ahead and have the Kit Kat at the movies," she advises. "If you don't satisfy an urge sometimes, you often substitute less-satisfying things and end up eating more." Her attitude is hard-won, and it came from educating herself about how to eat. "After I read *The South Beach Diet,* it made me much less prone to reach for the bad stuff," she says. So what's the good stuff? For breakfast, quinoa mixed with probiotic yogurt and sprinkled with raw oatmeal. For lunch, a salad with herbs, chopped tomatoes, and lentils, tossed with olive oil and vinegar. At dinnertime, "I'm cooking for two kids, and they don't think a dish is complete unless it's sitting on top of pasta!" Brinkley often swaps in healthier whole grain pasta, topped with sautéed or steamed vegetables. Add to that a protein source and a bean salad, and dinner is served.

Smile

It's one of the first things you notice about Brinkley: that smile. And it's very deliberate. "The mere act of putting your lips in that position tells your body to release chemicals that instantly make you feel better." Brinkley takes it one step further: "Share your smile with the world. It's a symbol of friendship and peace." She feels so strongly about it that she works with Smile Train (a charity that repairs needy kids' cleft lips and palates). And from smiling, she believes, happiness is just a step away. "The Dalai Lama said it best: 'Happy people don't want to go to war.' Talk about prevention!"

Protect Our Planet

The best way to do this: Go organic—and local—whenever possible. You're not just avoiding chemicals, you're also withdrawing your support from a system that dumps toxins into our food and water. "We cannot allow dispersants to be dropped all over the BP oil spill," she says. "Those chemicals are also getting into our food supply."

She's also launched a line of ecofriendly fabrics and posts "pictures of my garden or the beaches," with links to environmental groups, on her Facebook page (www.facebook.com/christie.brinkley).

Be in the Moment

"Our lives are changing every second," says Brinkley, "sometimes almost imperceptibly, sometimes suddenly and overwhelmingly." So get over trying to stop the process; instead, this veteran of crisis advises, "You constantly try—it's never easy—to live in the moment, because really, that's all you can count on." Being in the moment is the most effective method she has found to deal with overwhelming shifts in her life. Along with this knowledge: There's almost always a lesson somewhere if you're willing to look for it—and brave enough to learn from it. "I really believe in the old expression that what doesn't kill you makes you stronger. It's through adversity that you find the strength you never knew you had."

Surround Yourself with Nature

When Brinkley walks into her garden and sees the dewdrops on the grass and the way the light filters through the leaves, "it just fills your soul," she says. "We would be lost without places in nature to replenish our souls." It can be as humble as your own backyard or as grand as, well, the Grand Canyon. "We need to protect our wilderness areas and national parks. Everywhere you travel, you see blight, denuded mountains, logging. If people know what's going on, they'll become activists to safeguard those places."

Don't Think about Yourself

"If you're feeling stressed out or sad, helping someone else will change it all for you," says Brinkley. "It gives you a world perspective." And you don't have to be Christie Brinkley (or George Clooney or Angelina Jolie, for that matter) to have an impact, she says earnestly. "There are a million ways to help—by stuffing envelopes, forwarding an e-mail, donating as little as a dollar. The second you switch your focus to a meaningful cause, you're no longer thinking about your own pain, sadness, or anxiety. When you help someone else, your own fear disappears."

Be Grateful

"Count your blessings all day long," counsels Brinkley. When you do that, she believes, almost anything bad that comes your way falls easily down the list, with the exception of parents dealing with sick children. "But short of that," she says wistfully, "I think we can find perspective and gratitude everywhere."

PHOTO CREDITS

INDEX

Boldface page references indicate photographs. Underscored references indicate boxed text.